Vaccinated – dead

Histopathological
findings following
COVID-19 vaccination

The original German edition was published under the title
„Geimpft - gestorben. Histopathologischer Atlas der Corona-Impfschäden“

Co-authors: Michael Mörz, Helmut Luck

Translation: Dr. M.O. Gelin (Australia), Dr. Cordelia Kirchhoff-Stewens (Great Britain)
and Dr. Paul Brandenburg (Germany)

Translations of medical vocabulary and traditional jargon from one language to another can be challenging.
All efforts have been made to enable English speaking readers to fully
grasp the pathological findings made in the Institute in Reutlingen, Germany.

Corage Media
Imprint of Etica Media B.V., Swalmen, NL
For the English edition:

Layout: Martin Z. Schröder (Germany)
Typesetting: Gabi Gerhardt (Germany)
Printing and binding: Gyomai Kner (Hungary)
Printed in the EU – ISBN 978-9-083-52595-2

Etica Media – good, courageous and beautiful media with values
Contact: contact@etica.media
Website: www.corage.media

corage.media

Memorial publication for Prof. Arne Burkhardt

Vaccinated – dead

Histopathological findings following COVID-19 vaccination

UTE KRÜGER · WALTER LANG

corage.media

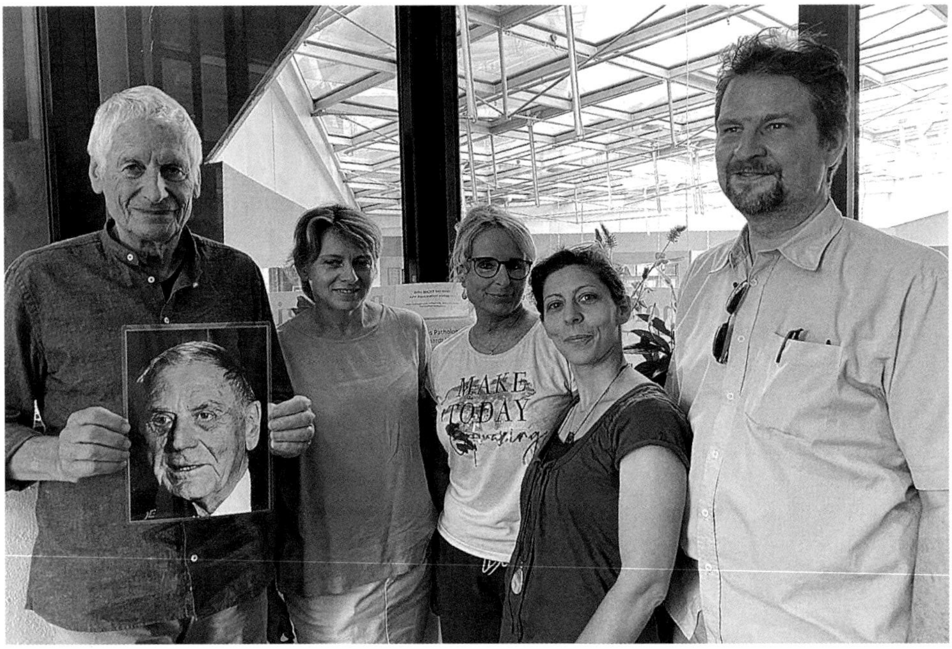

The staff of the Institute in Reutlingen, Germany, from left to right:
Prof. Walter Lang with the picture of Prof. Arne Burkhardt, Oksana Faul,
Ulrike Buschbacher, Enza Haider and PD Dr. Norbert Schwarz in September 2023
www.pathologie-konferenz.info

In memory of our dear and esteemed colleague

Prof. Dr. Arne Burkhardt,

whose many years of experience as a pathologist
and his tireless work and courage contributed to the creation
of this important and unique atlas

Table of contents

Foreword 9

Introduction (material and method) 11

General findings 15
1. Vasculitis 15
a) Vasculitis of large vessels 15
b) Vasculitis of small vessels 20
2. Thrombi 21
a) Classical thrombus 21
b) Fibrin thrombus 22
3. Substance deposits in the tissue 23
a) Amyloid-like deposits 23
b) Crystalline deposits of uncertain origin 24
4. Histopathologically visible phenomena 26
a) "Lymphocyte frenzy" 26
b) Spike protein detection 27
5. Destruction of elastic fibres 28

Organ findings 30
1. Heart 30
a) Myocarditis 30
b) Pericarditis 34
c) Deposits 36
d) Vascular changes 40
e) Ischaemic phenomena 44
2. Spleen 45
a) Vascular changes 45
b) Deposits 48
3. Liver 48
a) Inflammatory changes 48
b) Deposits 50
4. Brain 52
a) Inflammatory changes 52
b) Haemorrhages 53
c) Infarction 54

5. Lung 55
a) Inflammatory changes 55
b) Thrombi 56
c) Deposits 57
6. Thyroid gland 59
a) Inflammatory changes 59
7. Adrenal gland 60
a) Deposits 60
8. Kidney 62
a) Vascular changes 62
b) Deposits 63
9. Urinary bladder 64
a) Inflammatory changes 64
10. Testicles 65
a) Inflammatory changes 65
b) Spermatogenesis disorder 65
11. Prostate 66
a) Inflammatory changes 66
12. Pancreas 67
a) Deposits 67
13. Peripheral nerves 68
a) Inflammatory changes 68
14. Skeletal muscles 68
a) Inflammatory changes 68
b) Deposits 70

Case reports 71
1. Autopsies 71
2. Biopsies 127
3. Abortion 132

Summary of the findings 134

Conclusion 136

Acknowledgements 137

About the authors 138

Foreword

In the first few weeks of 2020, there was an avalanche of media reports around the world about a new dangerous respiratory infection, which, originating in China, spread rapidly around the world as a pandemic. It was named COVID-19 and triggered by a variant of an influenza virus from the well-known group of coronaviruses, SARS-CoV-2. Initial analyses, including those from the Diamond Princess cruise ship, indicated average infectivity, pathogenicity and mortality compared to other influenza viruses and did not confirm the initial fears. Nevertheless, a massive fear of an impending pandemic was created in almost every country in the world and, on this basis, measures such as border closures, exit restrictions, etc., which had previously been considered unthinkable and ineffective, were introduced. As there is no treatment for viral infections, all hopes were pinned on a vaccine that could be developed quickly. And in a very short time of less than a year, which was previously unthinkable, a vaccine was already available at the end of 2020. Due to the now widespread fear of the virus, supported by massive campaigns by most governments and constantly perpetuated by the media, around 70 % of the world's population subsequently had this vaccination administered at least once and often several times.

Only a few doctors and scientists issued warnings at the time. On the one hand, the vaccination had been completely inadequately tested, and the investigation, which normally takes at least 8 years until authorisation, had been shortened to a few months. On the other hand, the COVID-19 vaccination was a completely new technology that had never been used on such a large scale before. With previous vaccinations, a weakened or killed pathogen is injected and our immune system is ‚trained' by memorising the pathogen's recognition characteristics, the antigens. In the COVID-19 vaccination, however, a genetic code, mRNA is injected, which causes the body's own healthy cells to produce the recognition feature, the antigen of the SARS-CoV-2 virus. As a result of this misdirection, the immune system mistakes our own vaccinated body cells for a virus and destroys them. The disease symptoms triggered by this depend on the organ in which the cells were destroyed. And since the mRNA can infiltrate the cells of all organs, vaccination complications can also occur in all organs.

In other words, the COVID-19 vaccination causes an auto-immune response that has never been seen before. The symptoms of the vaccination complications are also new to medicine, which is why there is no experience of diagnosis and treatment. Unfortunately, there was also a widespread lack of interest among doctors in investigating these new phenomena.

In March 2021, lawyer Elmar Becker and pathologist Prof. Arne Burkhardt decided to investigate deaths following COVID-19 vaccinations to find out whether there was a causal link. In July 2021, pathologist Prof. Walter Lang joined the team, and the two pathologists subsequently carried out histological examinations at the Institute of Pathology in Reutlingen that were unique in the world. They were supported by pathologists from major clinics and universities in Europe.

Following the unexpected and tragic death of Prof. Burkhardt, Prof. Lang, with the help of pathologist Dr. Ute Krüger and other colleagues, summarized the valuable work of the pathology team in this atlas for the first time and thus made it accessible to a wider public. The aim is to continue Prof. Burkhardt's important work to better understand the pathomechanism of this new technology and thus hopefully also to improve the diagnosis and, above all, the treatment of complications resulting from mRNA injection. According to current medical and legal standards, this should have been done before authorisation and widespread use.

DDr. Christian Fiala

Introduction

Material and method

At Prof. Burkhardt's Institute of Pathology in Reutlingen, Prof. Burkhardt and Prof. Lang examined tissue samples from deceased persons whose deaths had occurred in connection with an mRNA vaccination against SARS-CoV-2, hereinafter referred to as COVID-19 vaccination for the sake of simplicity. They were supported in their work by several pathologists from large clinics and universities in Europe. The tissue samples were sent from forensic medicine institutes or pathology institutes. Autopsies were usually requested by the relatives of the deceased. Tissue samples from diseased patients were also sent in by dermatologists and oncologists.

In all cases, the aim was to be able to answer the question of whether there could be a connection between the death or the disease of the person in question and a performed COVID-19 vaccination.

The answers to this question were categorised into three groups:

Group 1 – a connection with a probability bordering on certainty
Group 2 – a probable or very probable link
Group 3 – no certain association

To our knowledge, the detailed analysis by the Burkhardt Institute, related to injuries that may have occurred in connection with mRNA vaccination was the only initiative of its kind in the world, which at the time, was seeking to understand the massively worrying complications caused by the completely new mRNA technology and to help develop both diagnostic options and therapies.

By June 2023, autopsy material from 89 deceased patients and biopsy material from 75 living patients had been analysed at the institute in Reutlingen. The cases mentioned, were numbered in the order in which they were received. One case documented in this atlas was examined at an institute in Sweden and is therefore labelled ‚external'.

In all cases, the specimens were examined using routine staining with Haematoxylin-Eosin (HE). Numerous special staining methods, such as Congo red, Iron and Elastika van Gieson (EvG) were used. Further immunohistochemical analyses were also carried out.

Immunohistochemical markers (antibodies) for identification of spike protein and nucleocapsid were used. If isolated spike protein was detectable in the tissue with a simultaneous negative reaction of SARS-CoV-2 nucleocapsid and with simultaneous tissue damage – then a reaction and/or damage due to the COVID-19 vaccination, could be assumed. Things became more complicated when there was a reaction to both the SARS-CoV-2 spike protein and the nucleocapsid. This reaction pattern indicated the presence of a COVID-19 infection, but logically this could not reliably rule out vaccine damage. The reason for this is simple: a vaccine-injured person can also have coronavirus, which means that both antibody reactions must be positive.

Only the histological sections of the case to be presented in the Atlas, for which a declaration of consent for publication had been obtained was available, were reviewed again and relevant sections were digitised and digital histological images were produced. Only individual specimens were examined under a light microscope and photographed in polarised light.

Unfortunately, the section thickness of the specimens, especially with regard to the special stains, did not permit high-quality digitisation. Therefore, images using routine staining are often shown in the atlas.

It was not uncommon to find deposits in the organs of the deceased that the pathologists had never seen in the 50 years of their working life prior to the start of the COVID-19 vaccinations. These deposits were analysed in other, more research-oriented institutes, using energy-dispersive X-ray spectroscopy, Raman spectrometry and laser microscopy. For the picture presented in this atlas, taken with the laser microscope, a tissue section stained with HE was used.

This atlas shows both strongly and discretely pronounced findings in order to draw attention to the grading of the findings.

The structure of the findings is based on the order suggested by Prof. Burkhardt. The first section shows only generally visible findings, which make the pathomechanism of the immune response triggered by the novel mRNA COVID-19 vaccination recognisable. In the second part, the various organs with the organ-specific damage are illustrated in detail. The numbering of the images is based on the table of contents. In addition, different patient cases were numbered consecutively for several cases in one category (e.g. in the chapter "General findings" for the category "1.a – Vasculitis of large vessels" there were five listed patient cases, which were labelled "Fig. 1a1" to "1a5").

Unfortunately, there were no submissions of material from deceased patients with malignancies that occurred relatively shortly after the COVID-19 vaccination. Dr. Ute Krüger, who has worked as a breast pathologist for more than 18 years, had already established in autumn 2021, that since the introduction of COVID-19 vaccinations, breast carcinomas were growing more aggressively and patients were younger than usual at the time of diagnosis. There were also more frequent recurrences and these aggressive tumours often caused patients to die within a very short time.

Finally: a noticeable increase in the incidence of other malignant tumours had taken place since the start of the COVID-19 vaccination. In Germany, for example, the Tumour registry shows an increased incidence of malignant melanomas.

Numerous oncologists worldwide point to an above-average increase in the incidence of malignant tumours since the COVID-19 vaccination was introduced.

In the case report section of this atlas, the cases were numbered in the order in which they were received as case 1 to case 164 (C1 – C164). Autopsies were listed first, then biopsies and finally an abortion. Not all cases examined in Reutlingen however are listed in the case report section of this book.

In order to provide a quick overview, age, sex, number and type of COVID-19 vaccinations administered and, in cases of death, the time span until death occurred after the COVID-19 vaccinations, were given in days in the first line (e.g. for case 1: "82y / f / 2x Mod / 75, 40" means the following: 82 years of age / female / two Moderna vaccinations, death occurred 75 days after the 1st and 40 days after the 2nd COVID-19 vaccination).

General findings

1. Vasculitis

a) Vasculitis of large vessels

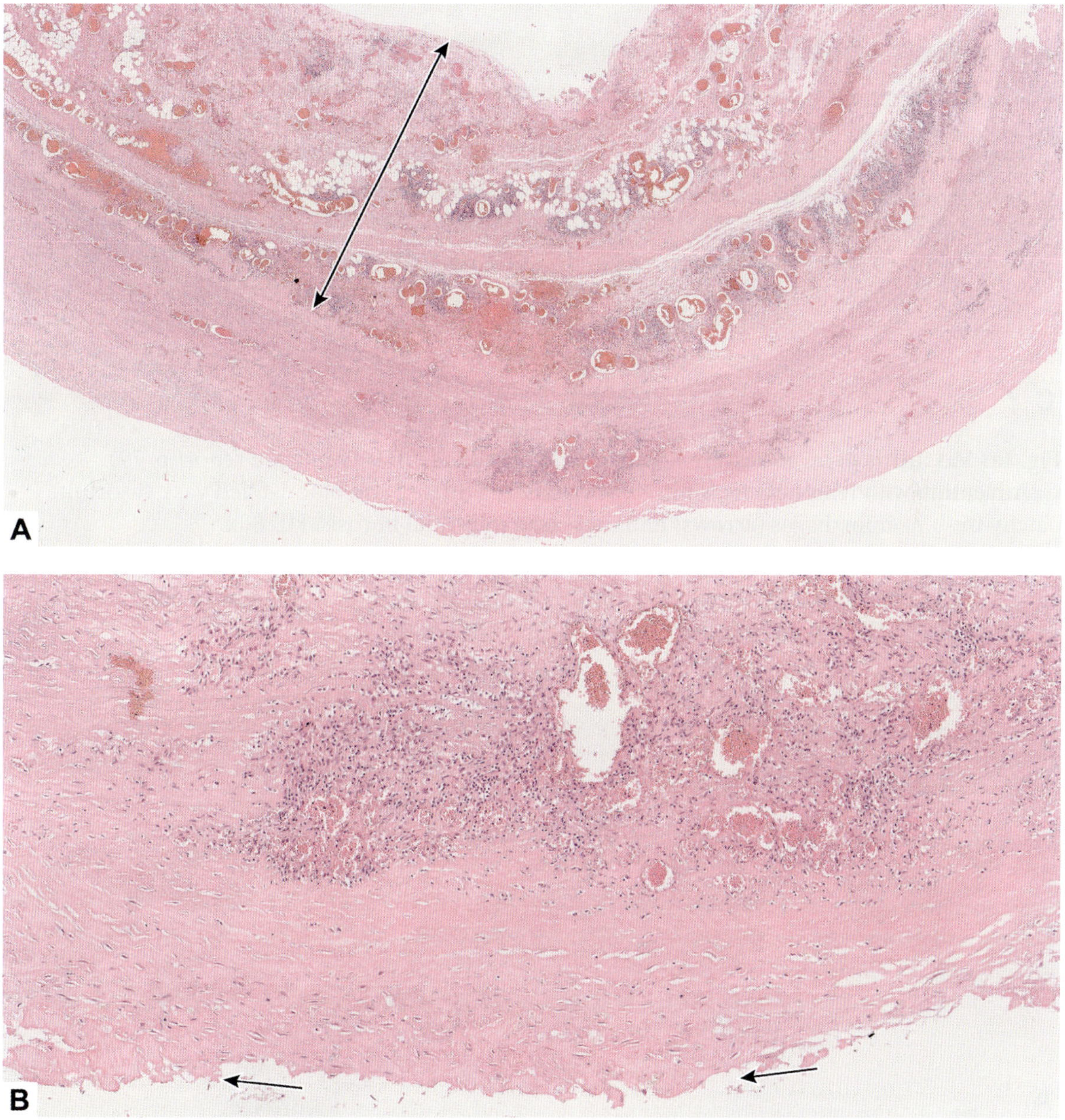

Fig. 1a1 Vasculitis of large vessels – Aorta: Case 10 (61y m, case report p. 79)
A: Aorta with marked wall thickening, conspicuous vascular proliferation in the wall, hyperaemia with patchy haemorrhage, lymphocytic infiltrates especially in the fibrotic adventitia (double arrow). HE 20x.
B: Degeneration of media with marked proliferation of the vasa vasorum and surrounding lymphocytic infiltrate. Intima forming an irregular luminal outline (arrows). HE 80x.

Continued on the next page.

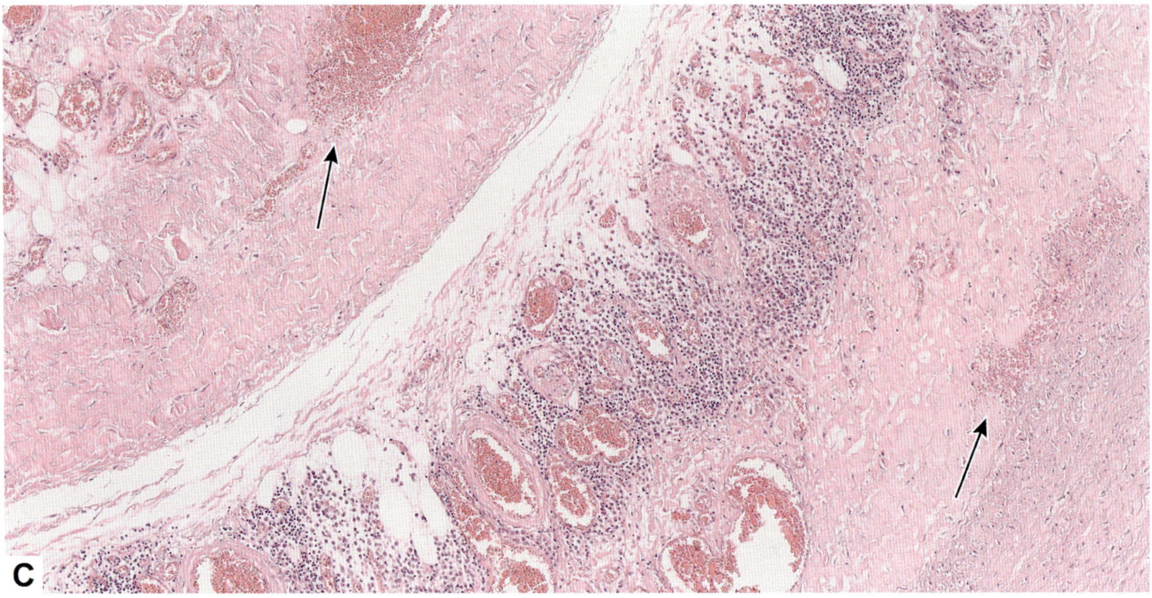

Fig. 1a1 Vasculitis of large vessels – Aorta: Continued case 10 (61y m, case report p. 79)
C: Adventitia with lymphocytic infiltrate surrounding dilated and blood-filled vasa vasorum, patchy fresh haemorrhages (arrows) and increased intestitial fibrosis. HE 80x.

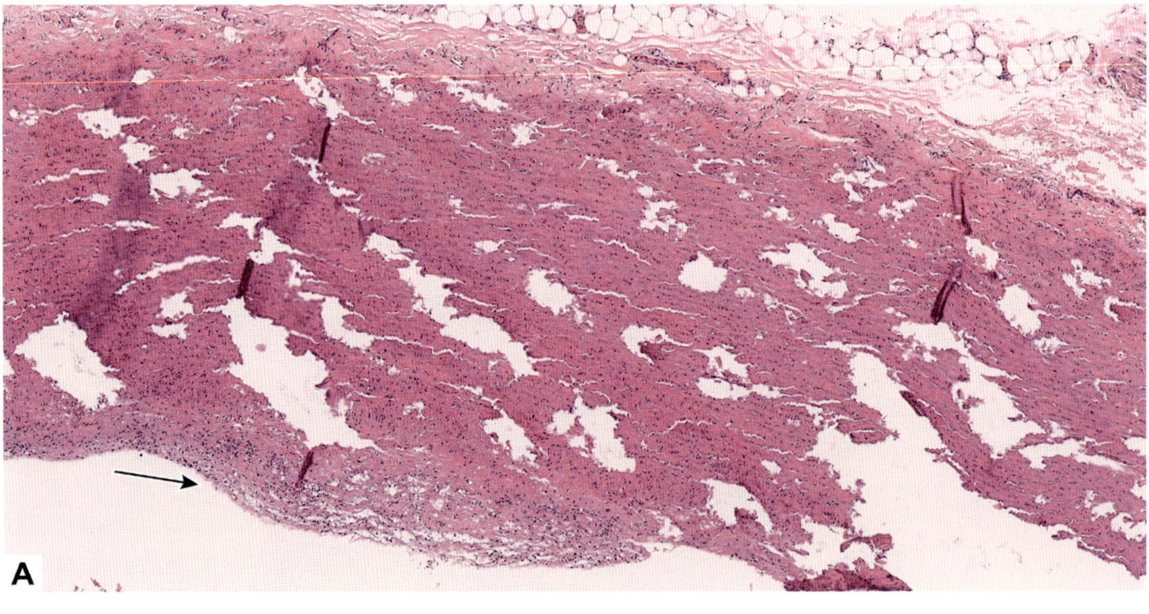

Fig. 1a2 Vasculitis of large vessels – Aorta: Case 66 (48y m, case report p. 103)
A: Despite cutting artefacts, easily recognisable cushion-shaped oedematous intimal thickening (arrow). HE 50x.

Continued on the next page.

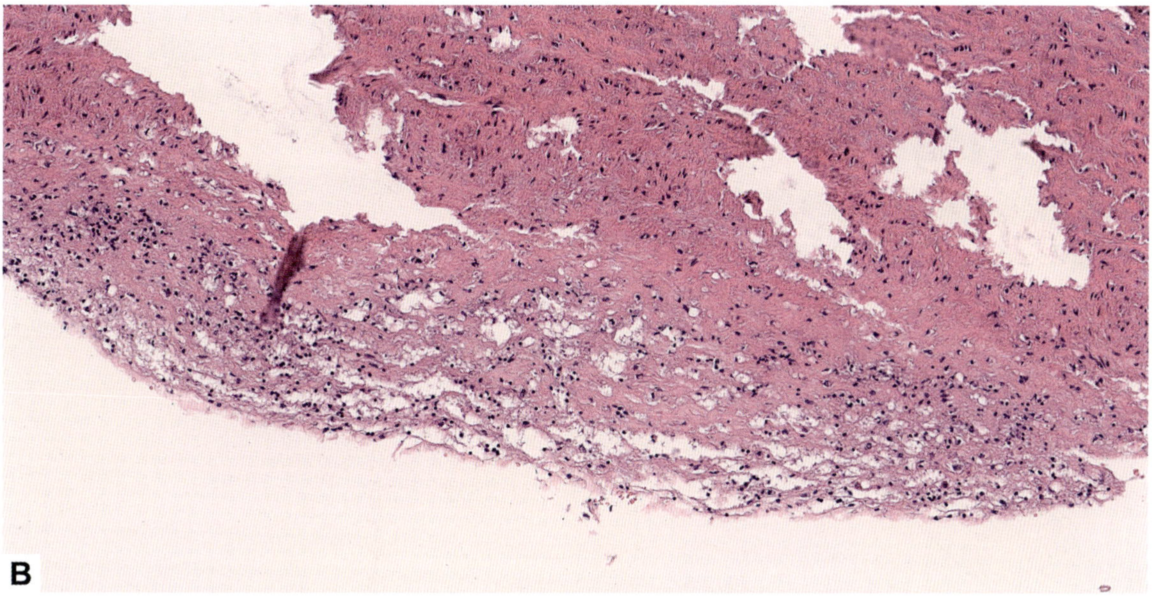
B

Fig. 1a2 Vasculitis of large vessels – Aorta: Continued case 66 (48y m, case report p. 103)
B: Cushion-shaped intimal thickening with oedema and lymphocytic infiltrate. HE 110x.

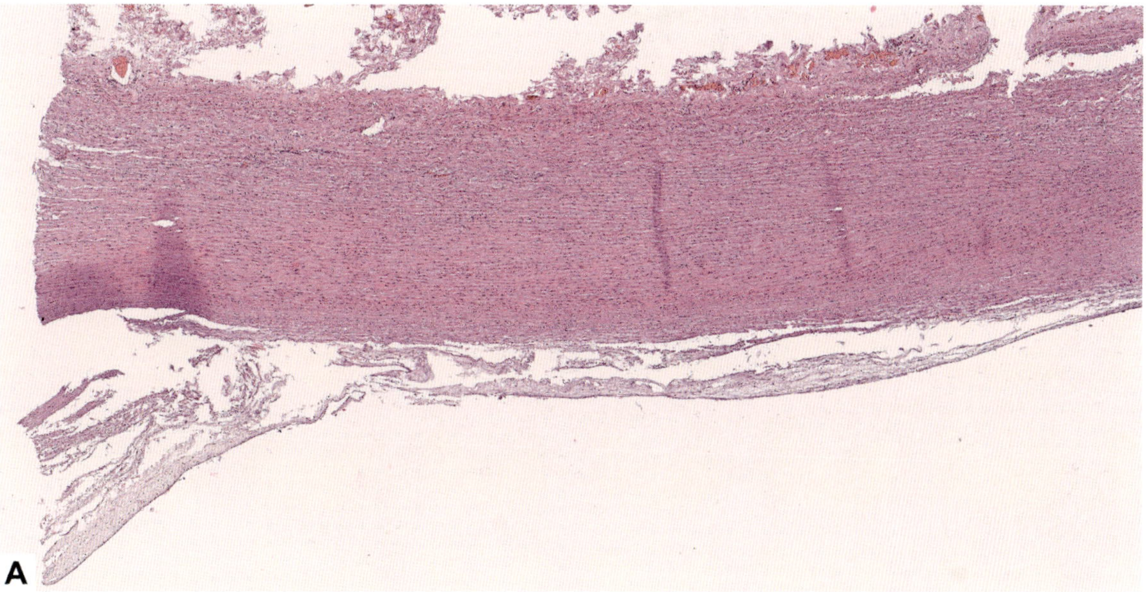
A

Fig. 1a3 Vasculitis of large vessels – Aorta: Case 42 (84y f, case report p. 94)
A: Oedematous intima. HE 30x.

Continued on the next page.

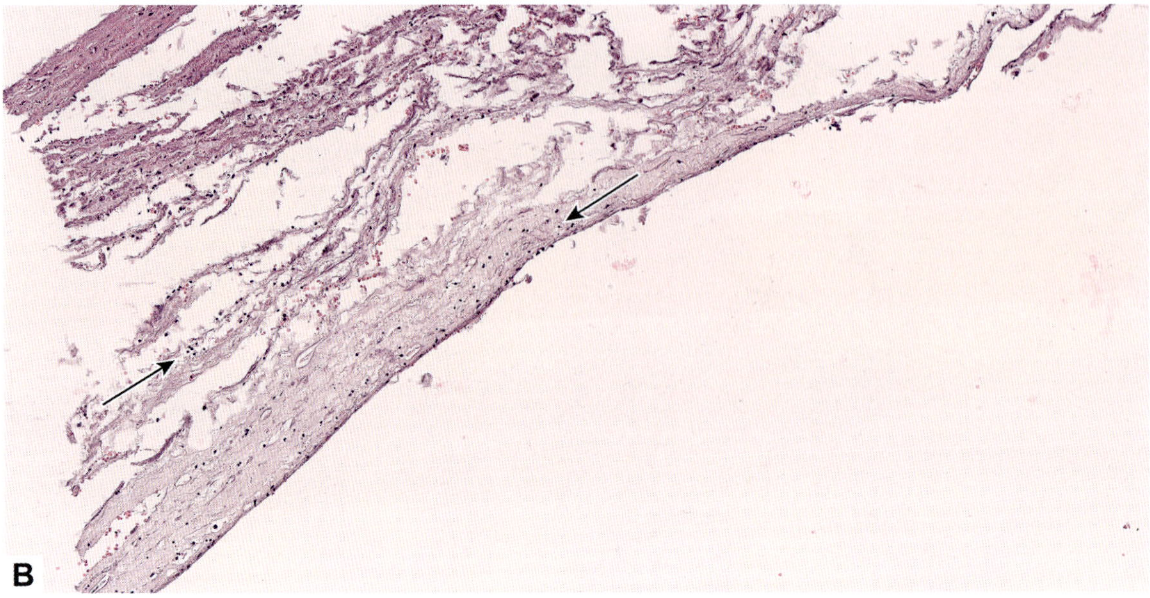

Fig. 1a3 Vasculitis of large vessels - Aorta: Continued case 42 (84y f, case report p. 94)
B: Intima oedematously loosened and with sparse inflammatory lymphocytic infiltrate (arrows). HE 100x.

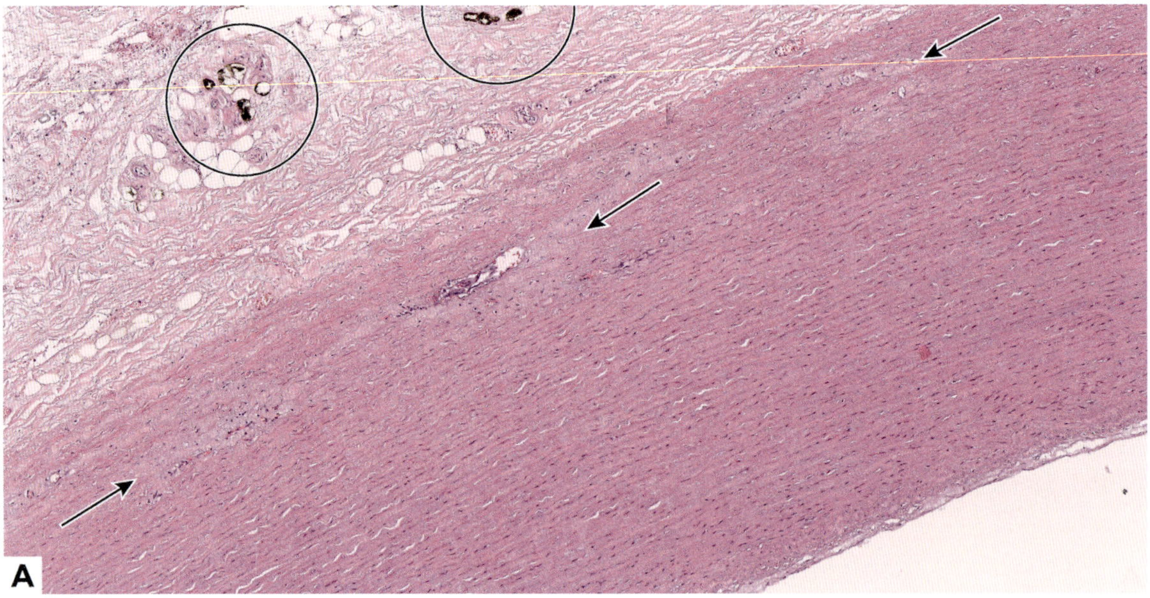

Fig. 1a4 Vasculitis of large vessels – Aorta: Case 46 (29y m, case report p. 95)
A: Degeneration of media with structural distortion of the deep wall layers (arrows) and proliferation of the vasa vasorum already recognisable in the overview. Intima slightly oedematously loosened. Crystalloid deposits of uncertain origin in the adventitia (circles). HE 60x.

Continued on the next page.

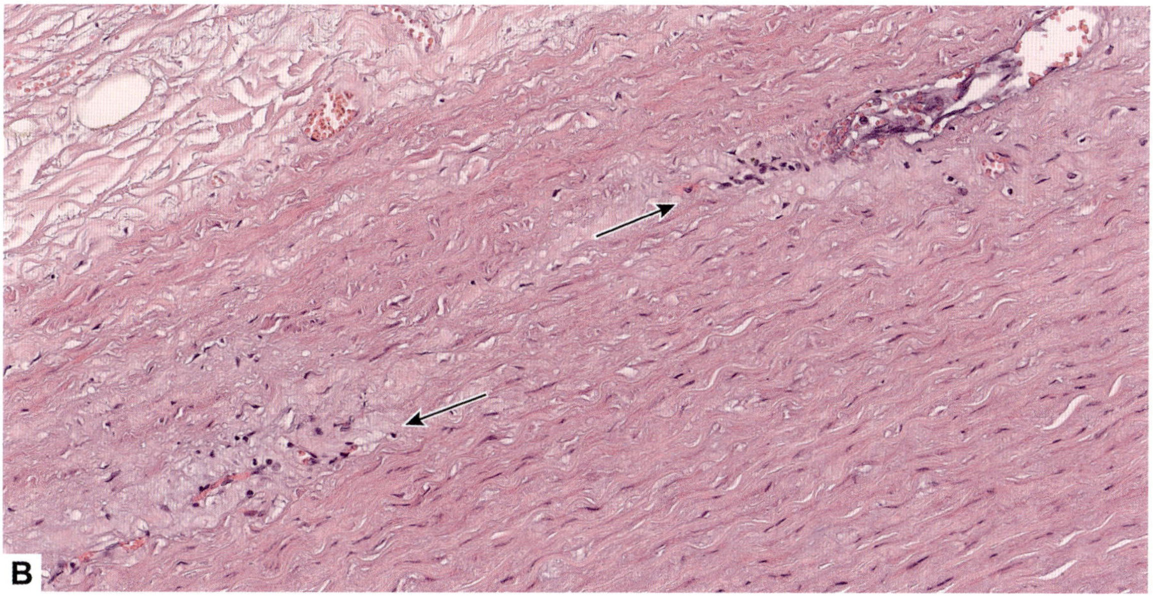

Fig. 1a4 Vasculitis of large vessels– Aorta: Continued case 46 (29y m, case report p. 95)
B: Loosening of the deep wall layers (arrows) with proliferation of the vasa vasorum, occasional lymphocytes. HE 160x.

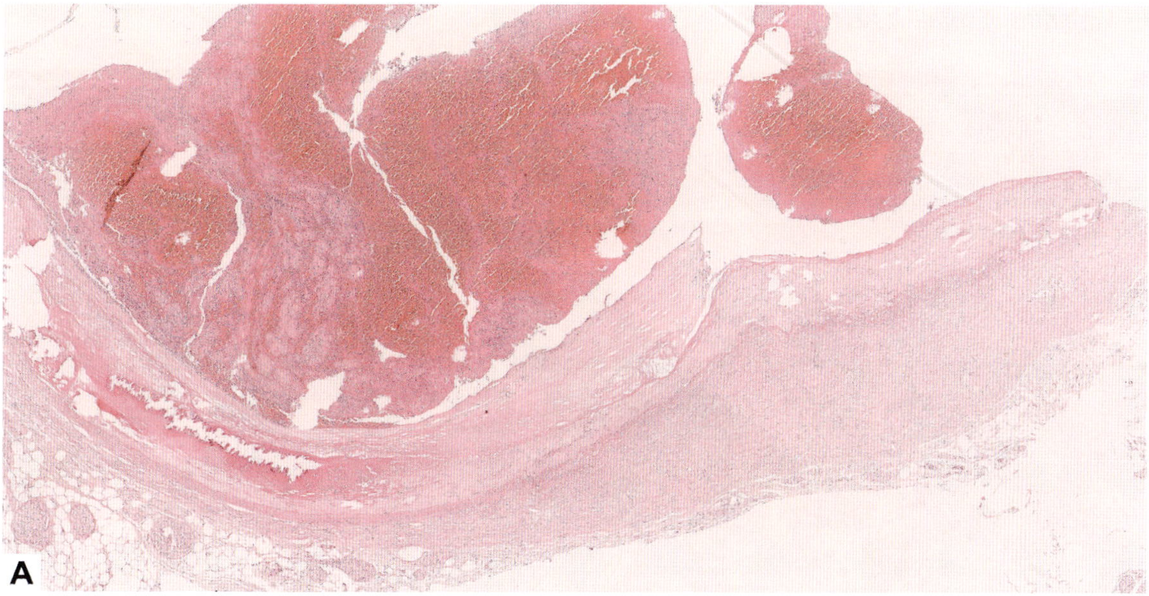

Fig. 1a5 Vasculitis of large vessels – Aorta: Case 9 (89y f, case report p. 78)
A: A. mesenterica superior, atherosclerotic pre-damaged, with clear intimal fibrosis, partially calcified plaques and acute layered thrombus in the lumen. HE 20x.

Continued on the next page.

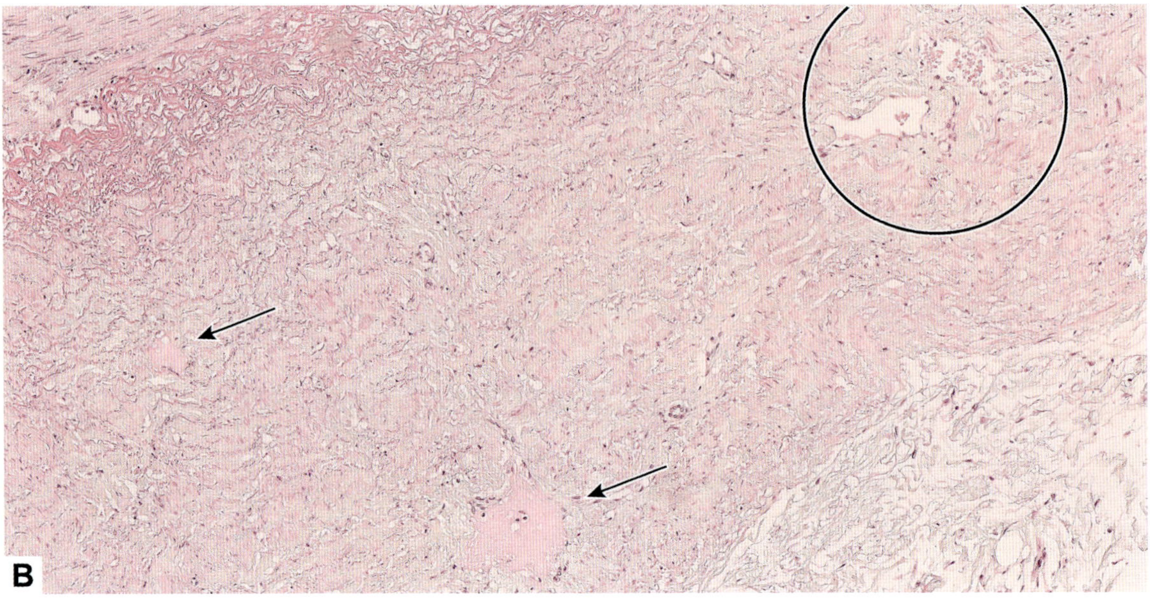

Fig. 1a5 Vasculitis of large vessels – Aorta: Continued case 9 (89y f, case report p. 78)
B: Media necrosis with loosened fibrous scaffold in numerous places, oedema in places (arrows) and sprouting of the vasa vasorum (circle). HE 90x.

b) Vasculitis of small vessels

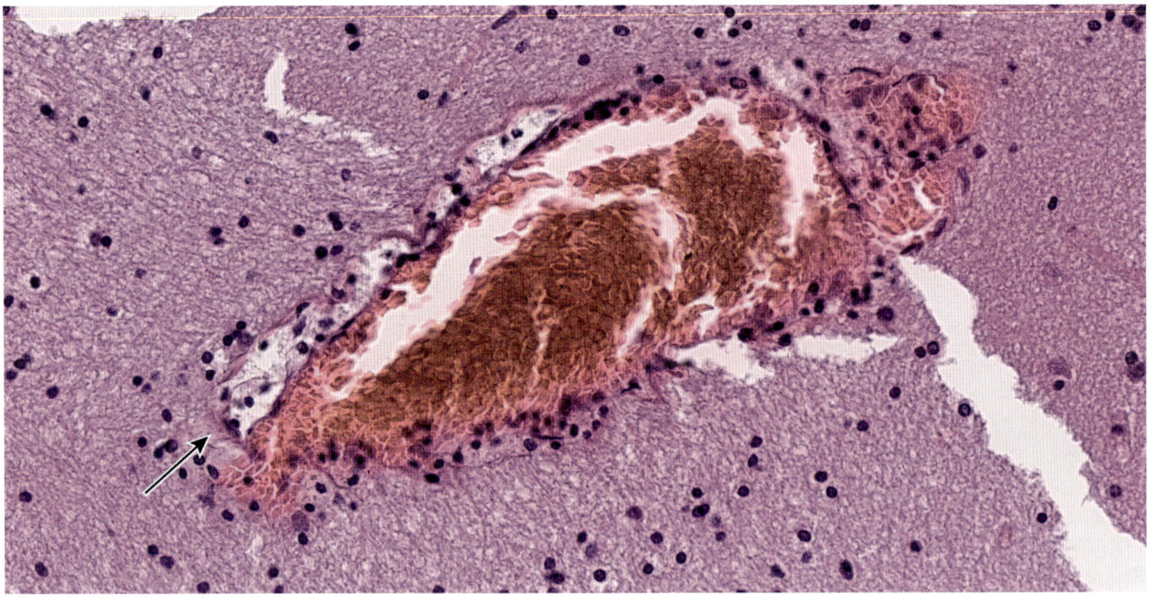

Fig. 1b Vasculitis of small vessels – Brain: Case 30 (39y m, case report p. 90)
Small calibre cerebral vessel with patchy but clearly visible oedema of the vessel wall (arrow) and lymphocytic infiltrate. HE 300x.

2. Thrombi

a) Classical thrombus

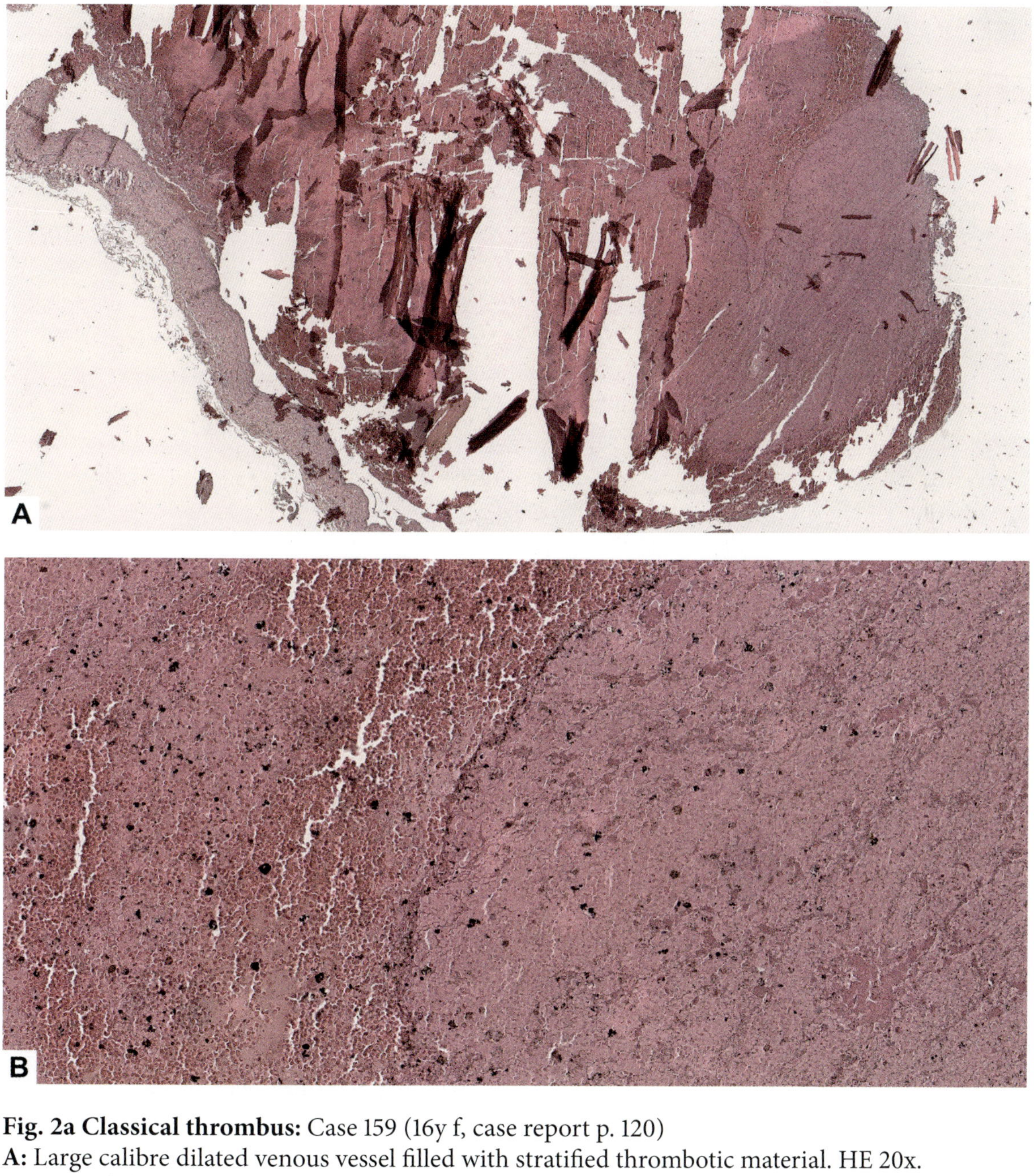

Fig. 2a Classical thrombus: Case 159 (16y f, case report p. 120)
A: Large calibre dilated venous vessel filled with stratified thrombotic material. HE 20x.
B: Layered thrombotic material consisting of a combination of red blood cells and fibrin. HE 100x.

b) Fibrin thrombus

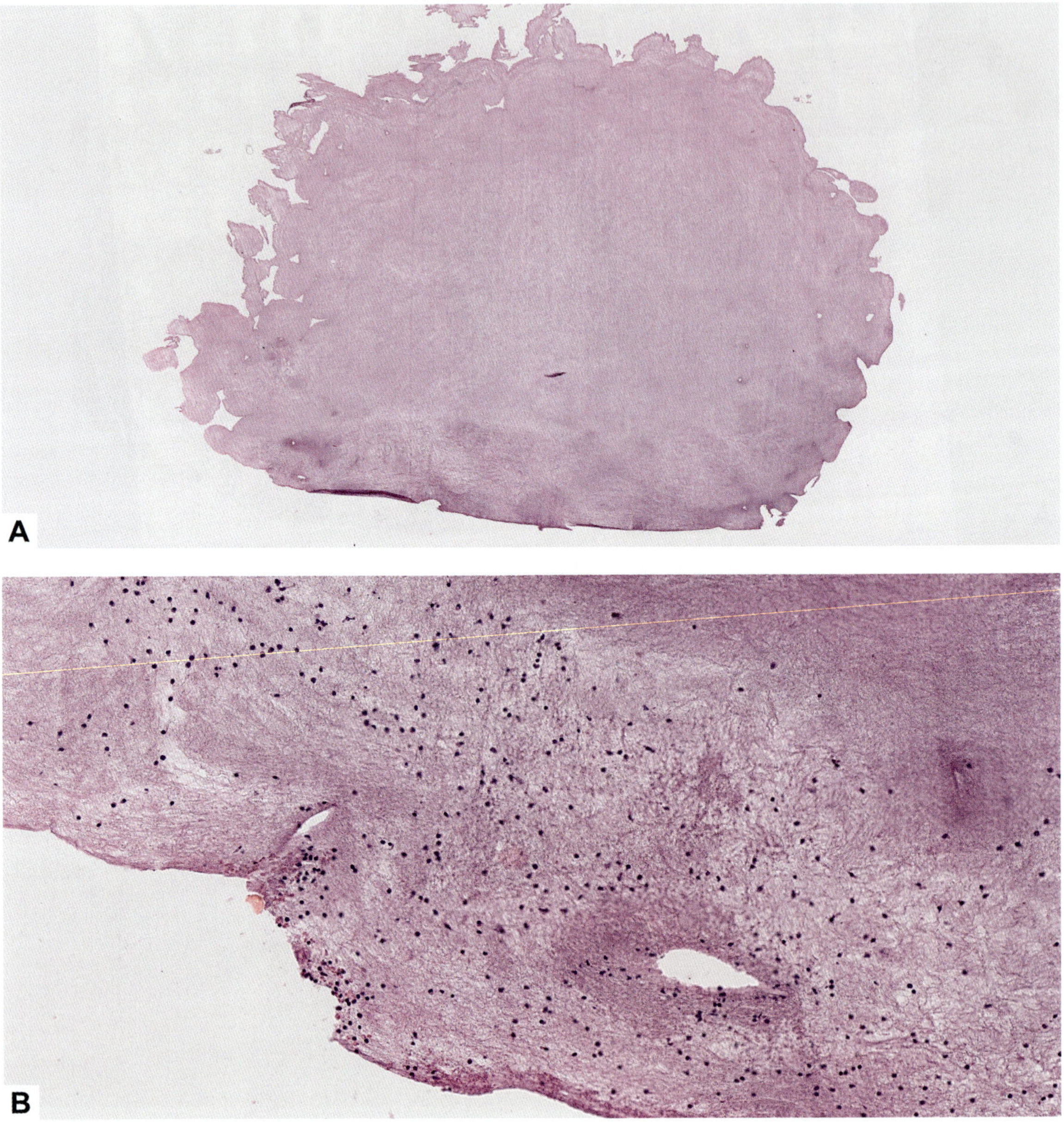

Fig. 2b Fibrin thrombus: Case 39B (43y f, case report p. 127)
A: Almost homogeneous material without detectable layering. HE 10x.
B: Fibrillar material without recognisable erythrocytes with loose lymphocytic infiltrate in places. HE 140x.

3. Substance deposits in the tissue

a) Amyloid-like deposits

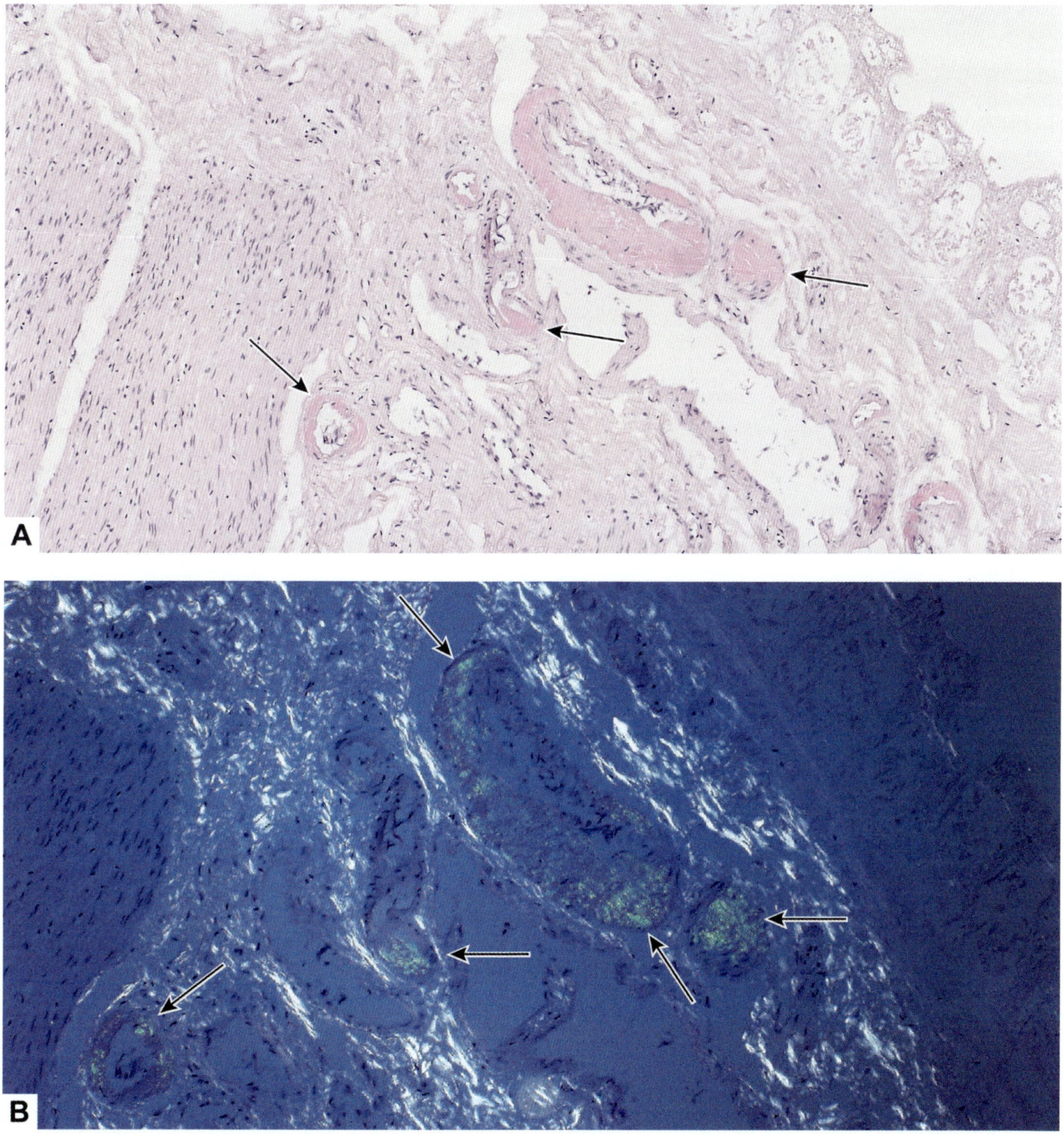

Fig. 3a Amyloid-like deposits – Colon: Case 3 (94y f, case report p. 74)
A: Submucosa with homogeneous, strongly eosinophilic-coloured material in numerous vessel walls (arrows), partly arranged in a circular pattern, with in some cases marked thickening of the vessel wall. HE 100x.
B: Already in routine staining in polarised light birefringent, clearly green shimmering material (arrows). HE 100x.

b) Crystalline deposits of un uncertain origin

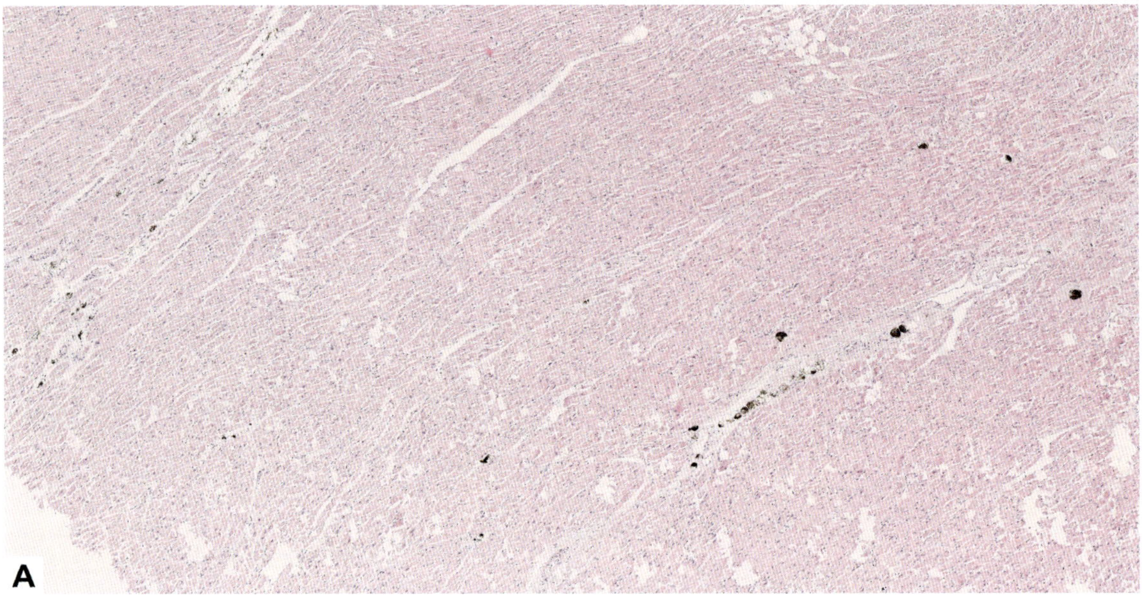

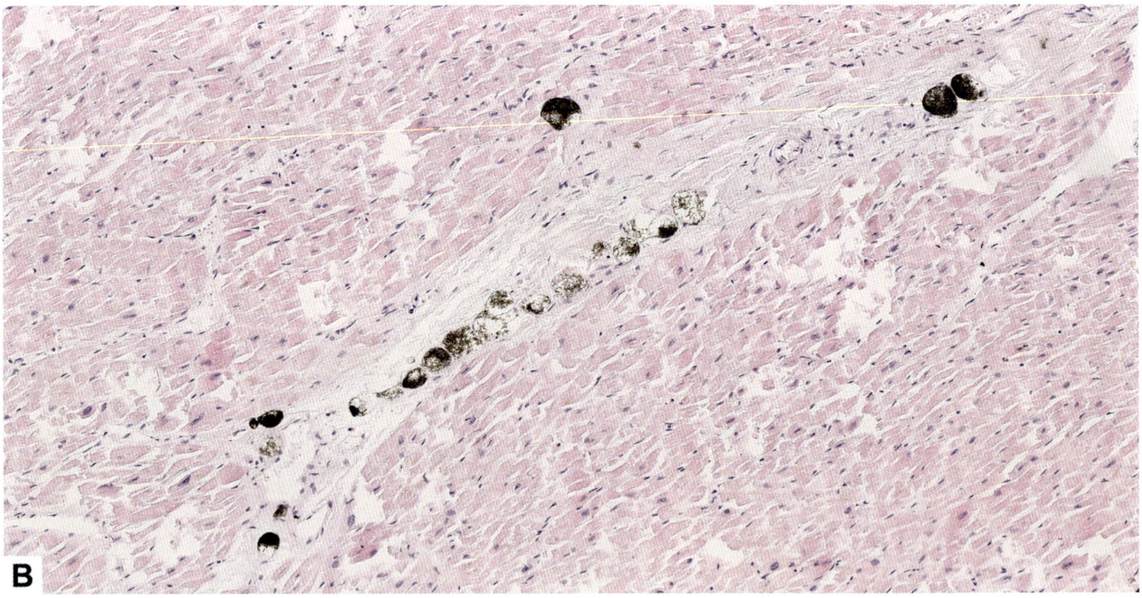

Fig. 3b Crystalline deposit of uncertain origin – Myocardium: Case 17 (83y f, case report p. 82)
A: Black crystalline deposits of uncertain origin found in numerous places in the interstitium. HE 20 x.
B: Black material apparently lying in adipocytes. HE 100x.

Continued on the next page.

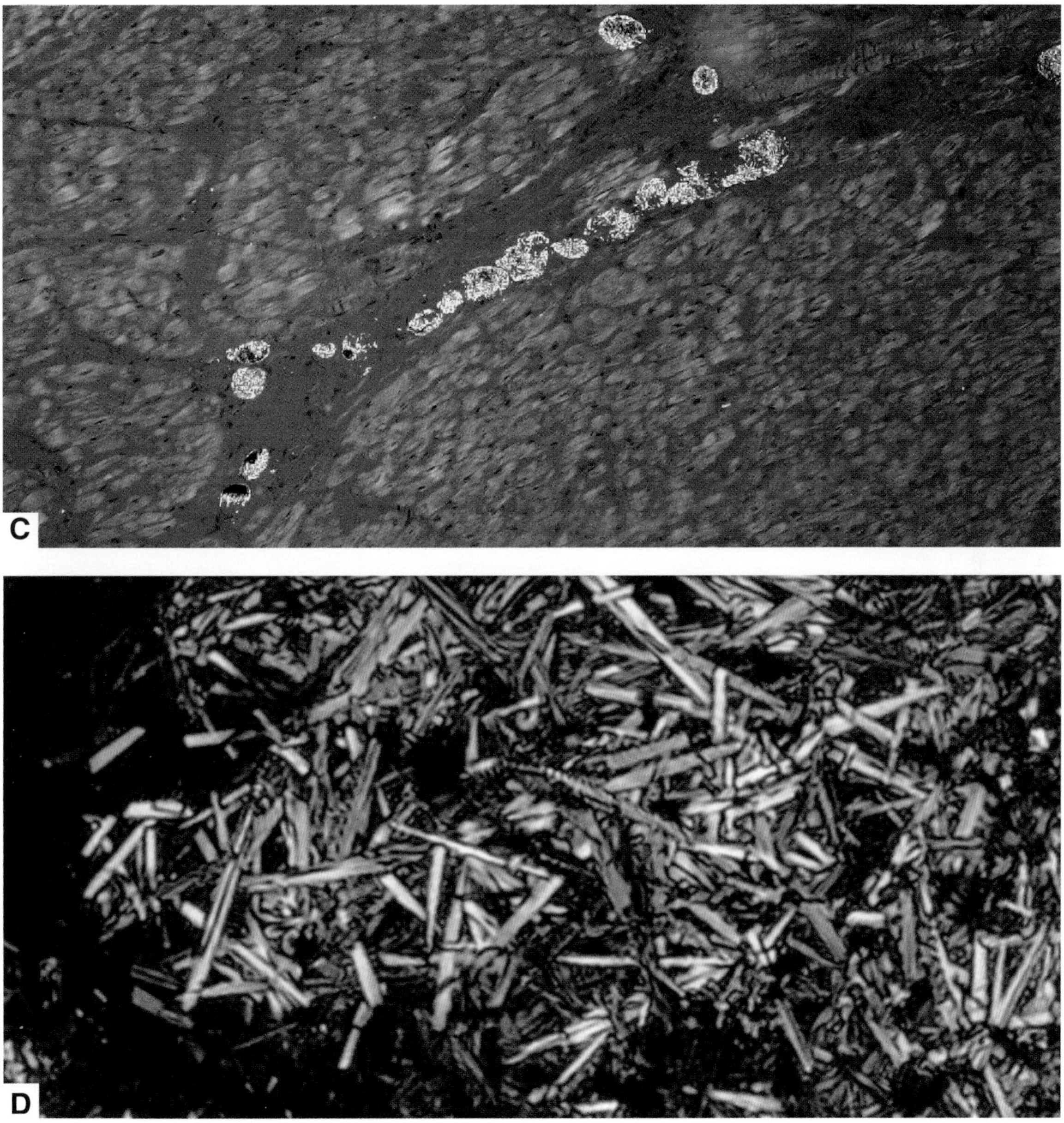

Fig. 3b Crystalline deposit of uncertain origin – Myocardium: Continued case 17 (83y f, case report p. 82)
C: In polarised light clearly birefringent material. HE 100x.
D: In the laser microscope visible, needle-shaped formations with often corkscrew-like ends. 6000x.

4. Histopathologically visible phenomena

a) "Lymphocyte frenzy"

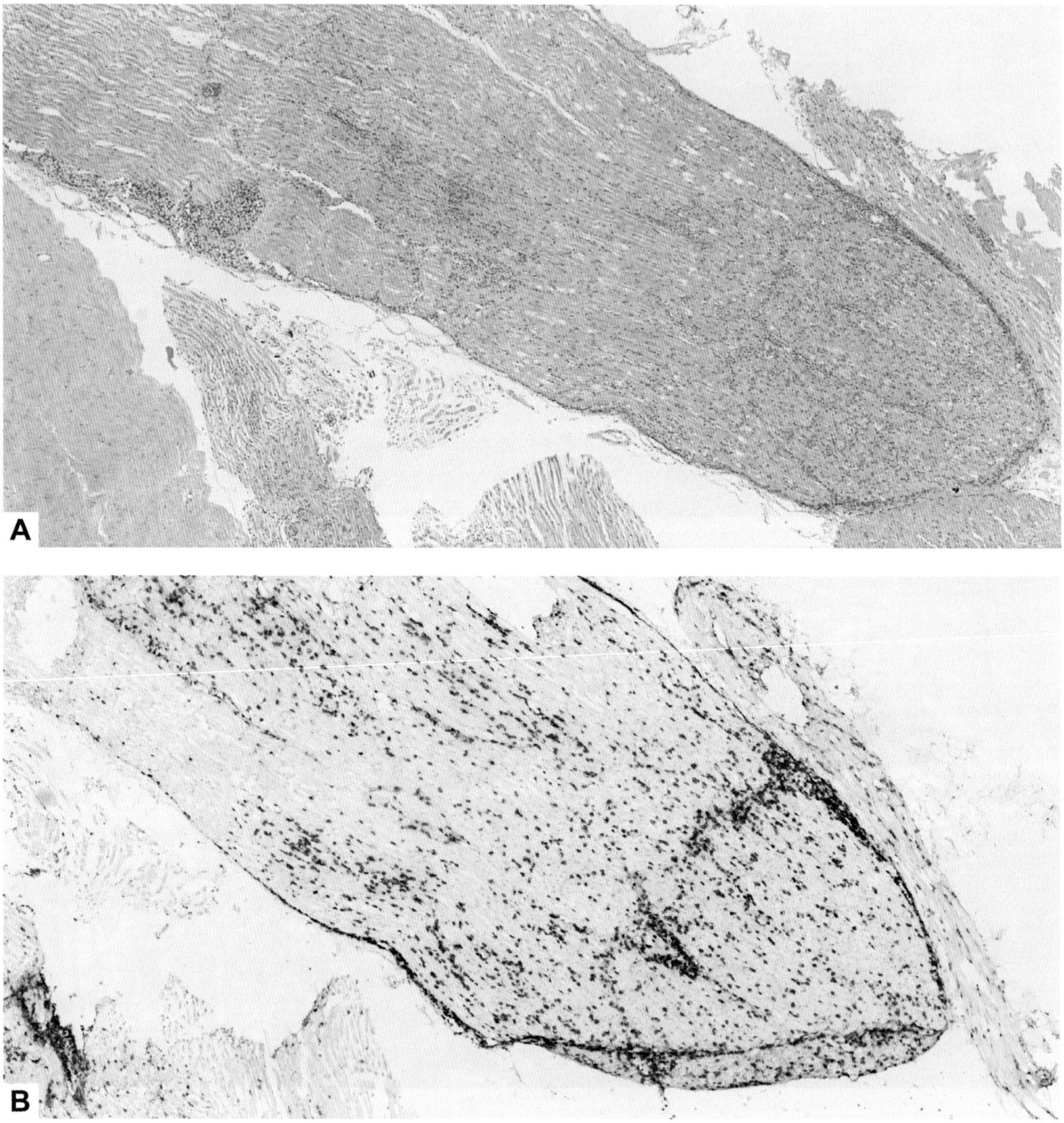

Fig. 4a "Lymphocyte frenzy" – Radicular nerve: external case (61y m, case report p. 125)
A: Dense lymphocytic infiltration, mainly intraneural. HE 50x.
B: Immunohistological positivity for the marker CD3, consistent with lymphocytes. CD3 70x.

b) Spike protein detection

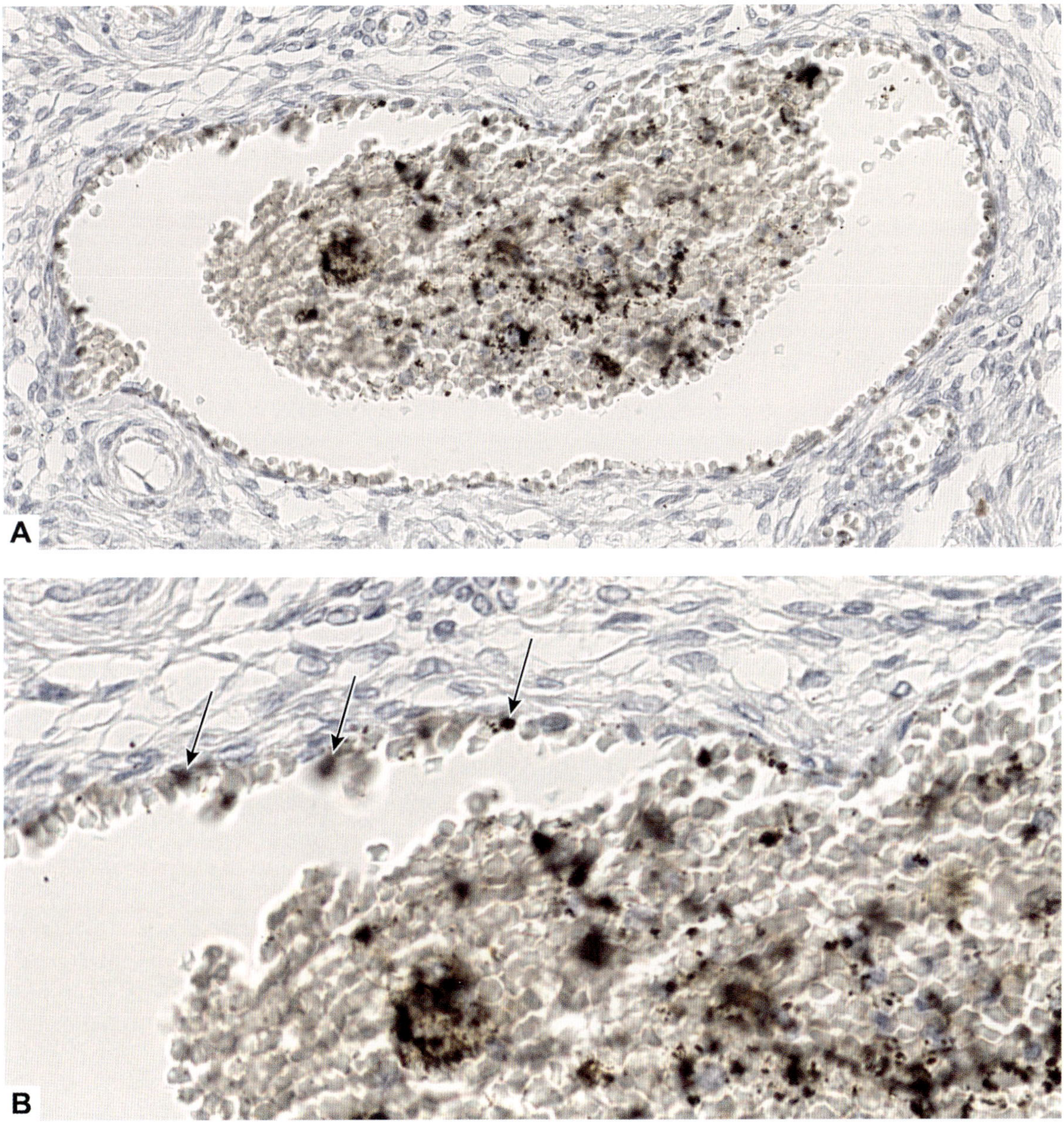

Fig. 4b Spike protein detection – Ovary: Case 159 (16y f, case report p. 120)
A: Ovary with dilated blood vessels and specific staining of the immunohistochemical marker. Spike protein 400x.
B: Positivity also in individual endothelial cells (arrows). Spike protein 600x.

5. Destruction of elastic fibres

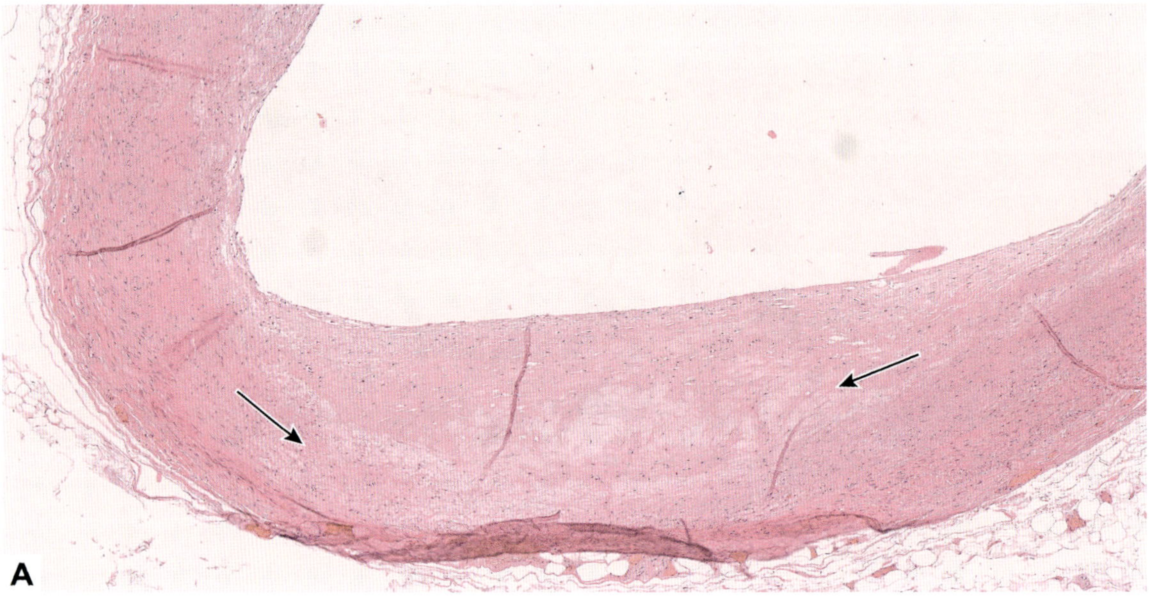

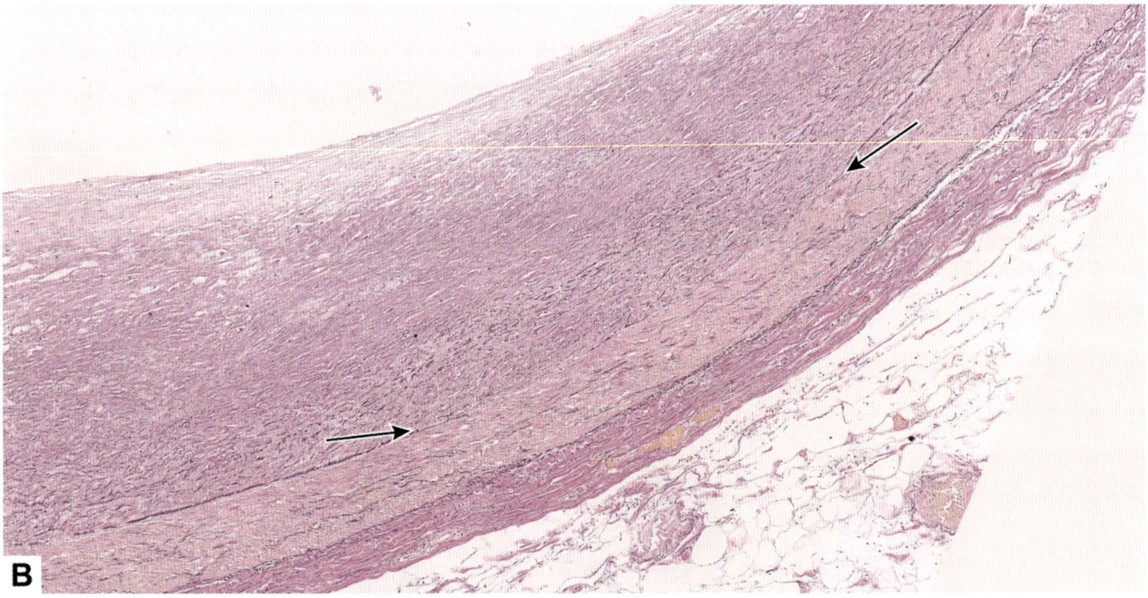

Fig. 5.1 Destruction of elastic fibres – Coronary artery: Case 91 (74y m, case report p. 111)
A: Atherosclerotic pre-damaged vessel with intimal thickening. Significant oedematous loosening of both the media and the intimal plaques (arrows). HE 40x.
B: Degeneration of media with loss of elastic fibres (arrows). EvG 80x.

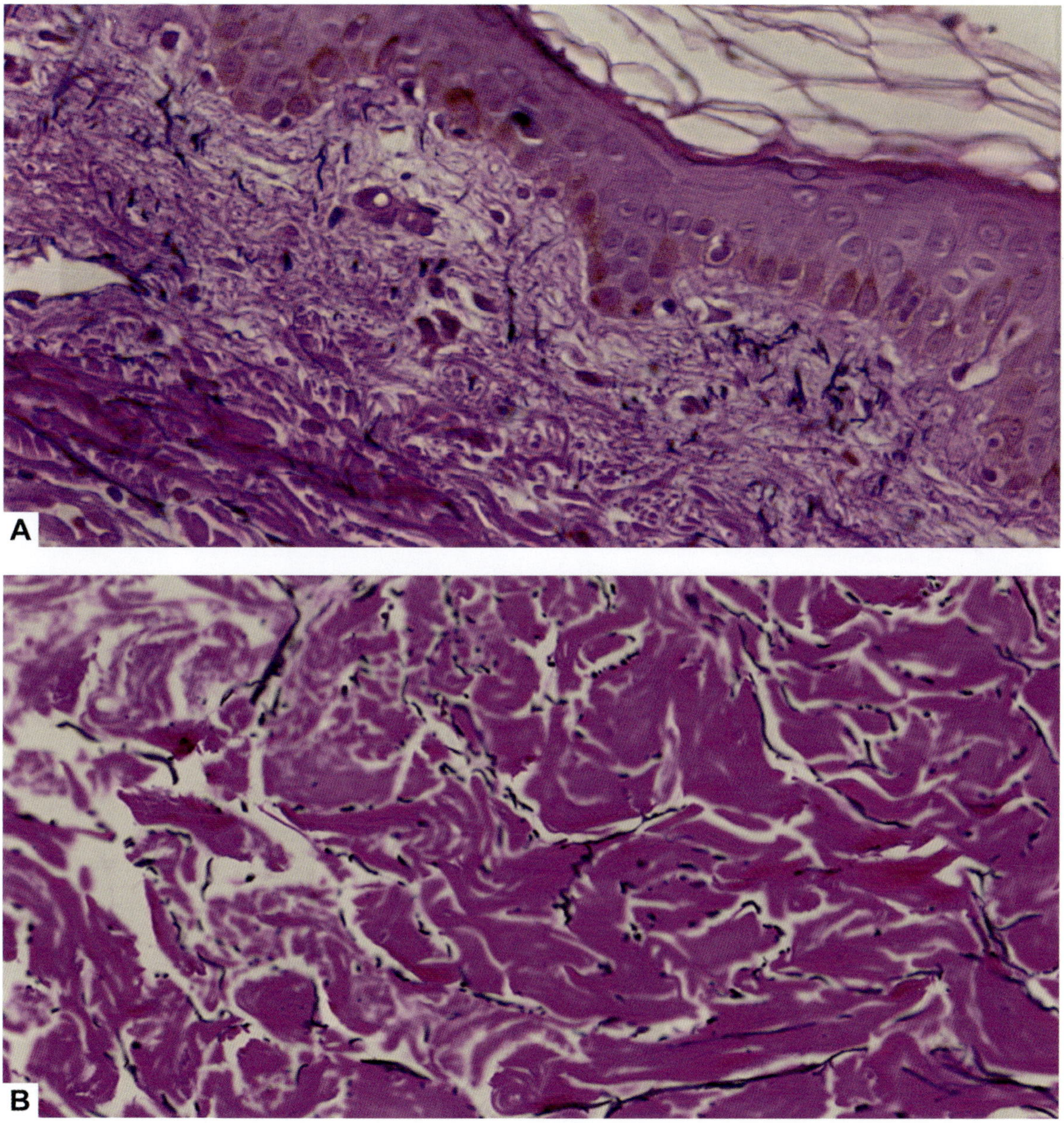

Fig. 5.2 Loss of elastic fibres – Skin: Case 113B (38y m, case report p. 129)
A: Significant rarefaction of the basement membrane-associated elastic fibres. EvG 150x.
B: Disruption and fragmentation of the elastic fibers within the deeper dermis. EvG 150x.

Organ findings

1. Heart

a) Myocarditis

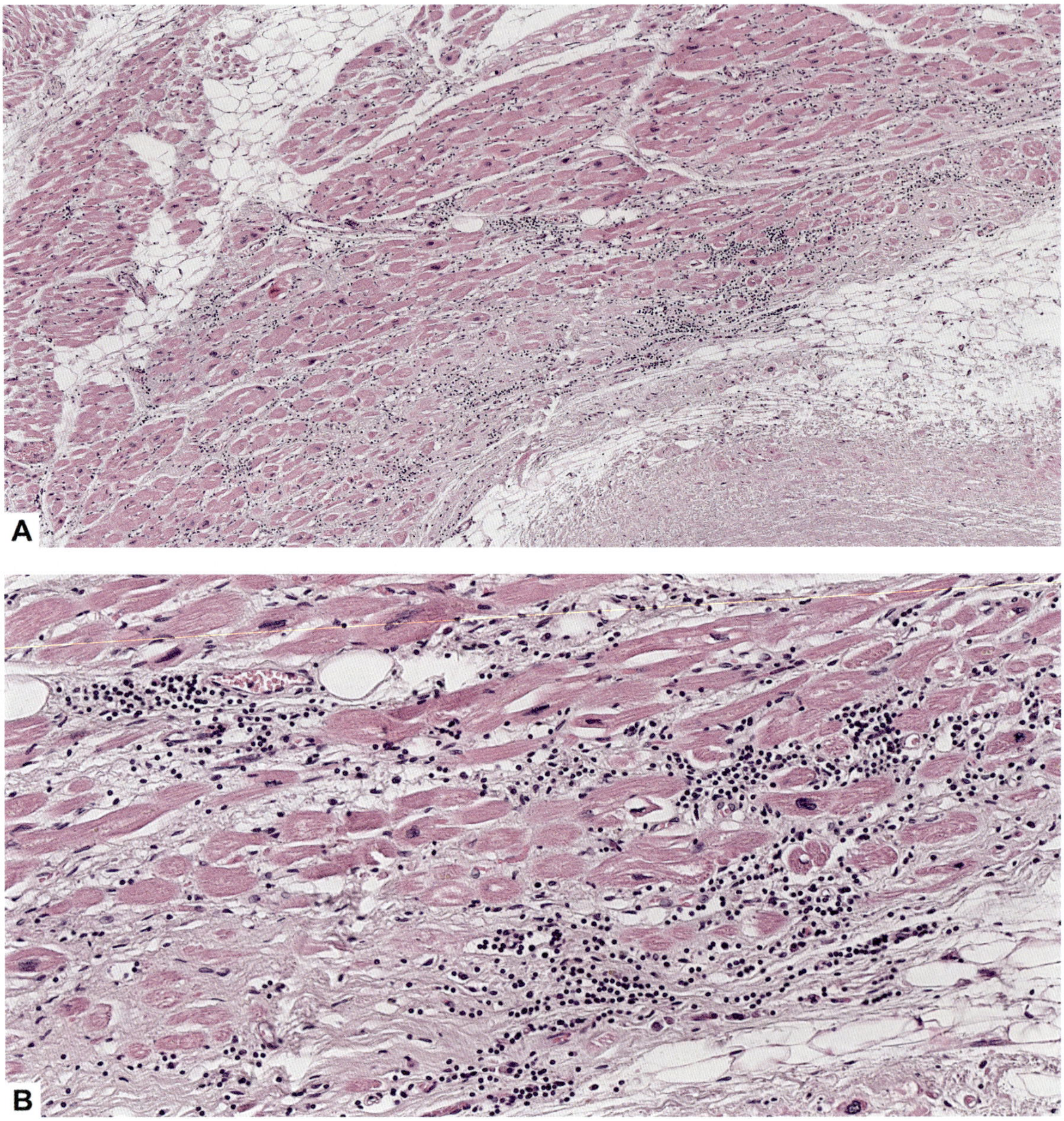

Fig. 1a1 Heart – Myocarditis: Case 56 (85y m, case report p. 98)
A: Patchy, partially dense lymphocytic infiltrate, interstitial scars. Enlarged cardiomyocyte nuclei. HE 60x.
B: Interstitial lymphocytic infiltrate and loose scar tissue, indicating a multistage process of myocarditis. Variation of size of cardiomyocyte nuclei. HE 200x.

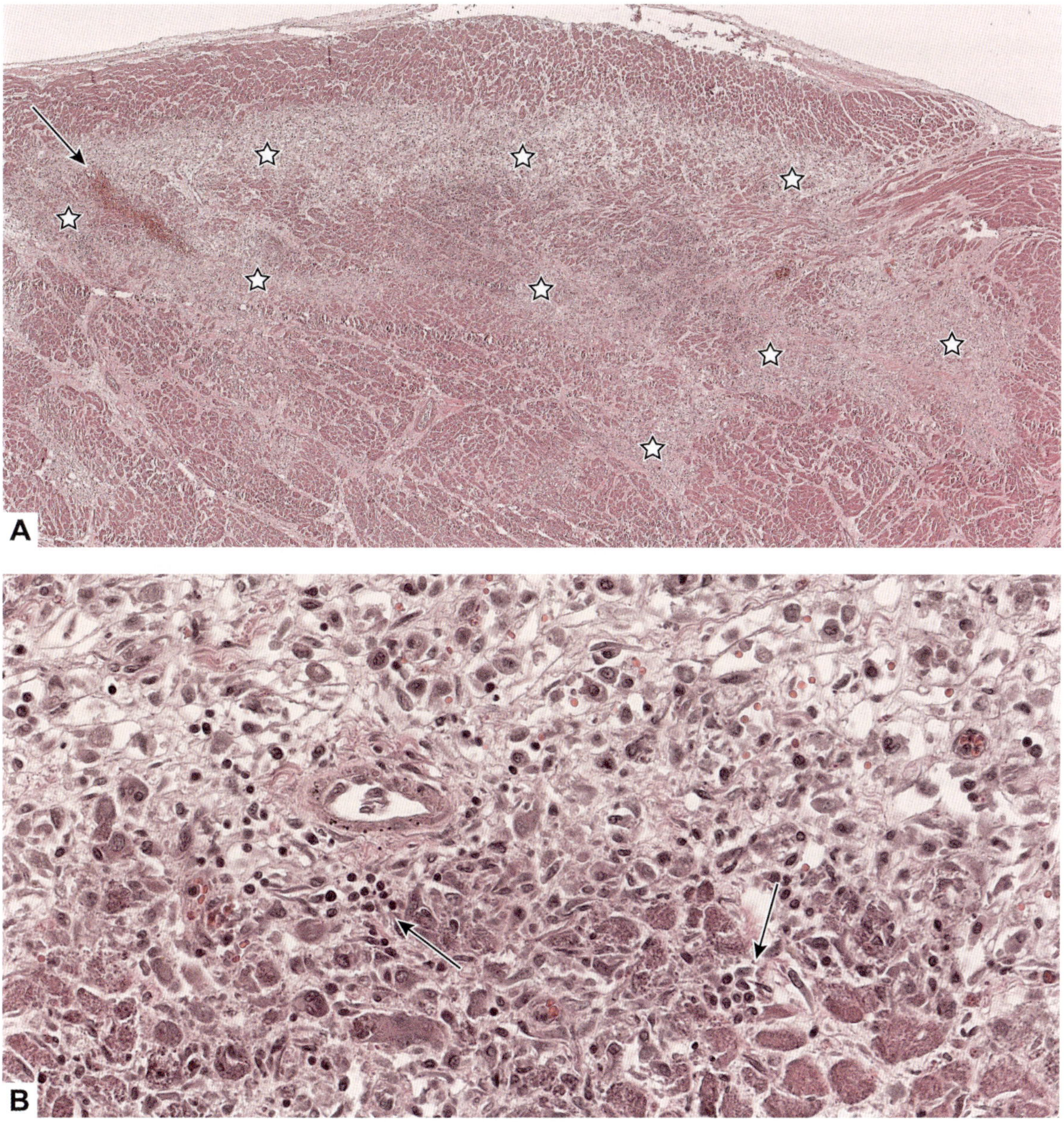

Fig. 1a2 Heart – Myocarditis: Case 159 (16y f, case report p. 120)
A: Myocardium with oedema, extensive necrosis and incipient loose scarring (asterisks) as well as focal fresh haemorrhage (arrow). HE 20x.
B: Visible atrophy of cardiomyocytes, localised infiltration with lymphocytes (arrows) and loose scarring in the upper part of the image, consistent with active chronic myocarditis. HE 300x.

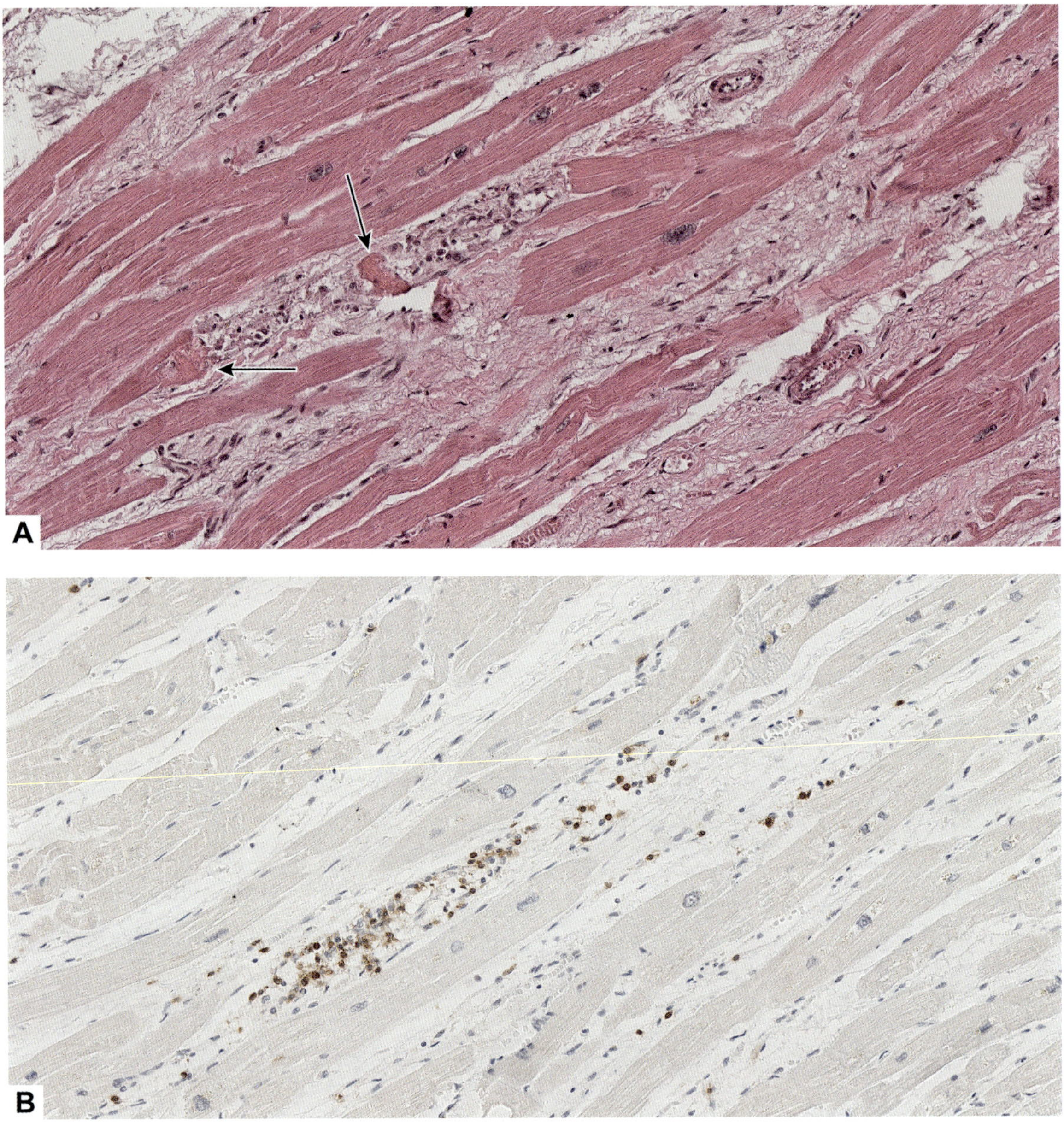

Fig. 1a3 Heart – Myocarditis: Case 111 (40y m, case report p. 115)
A: Myocardium with interstitial fibrosis, focal inflammatory infiltration and residual necrotic hypereosinophilic cardiomyocytes (arrows). HE 300x.
B: Patchy lymphocytic infiltrate with positivity for CD3, consistent with T cells. CD3 300x.

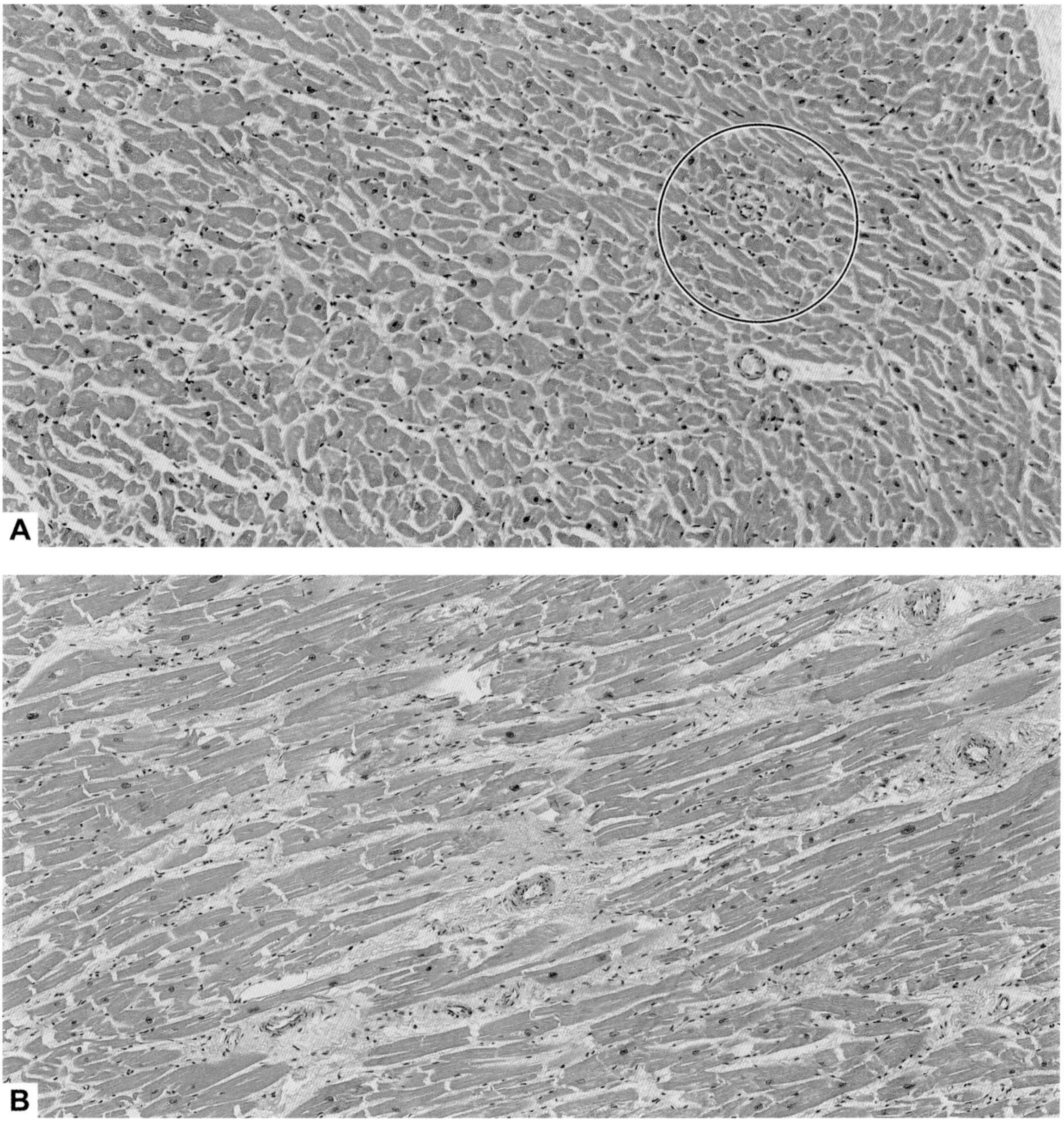

Fig. 1a4 Heart – Features of myocarditis: Case 85 (22y m, case report p. 110)
A: Minimally increased interstitial cell content (circle) and oedematous myocardium. HE 100x.
B: Spotty mild perivascular fibrosis, the image is compatible with residual myocarditis. HE 80x.

b) Pericarditis

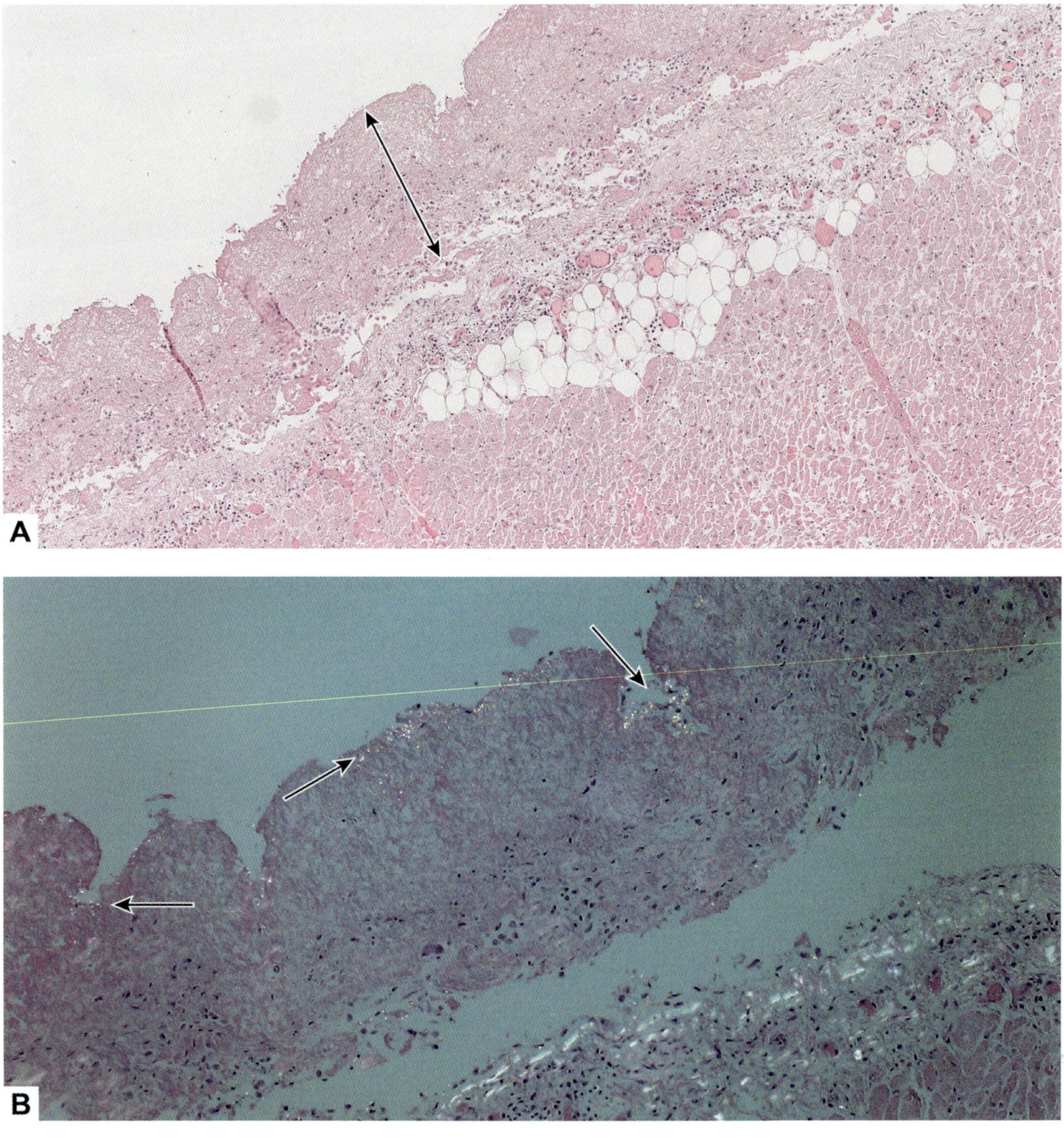

Fig. 1b1 Heart - Pericarditis: Case 21 (85y m, case report p. 87)
A: Pronounced fibrinous pericarditis with thick fibrin layer (double arrow) and subpericardial, band-like lymphocytic infiltrate. HE 60x.
B: In polarised light, birefringent crystalline material of uncertain origin in the upper layers of the fibrin layer (arrows). HE 100x.

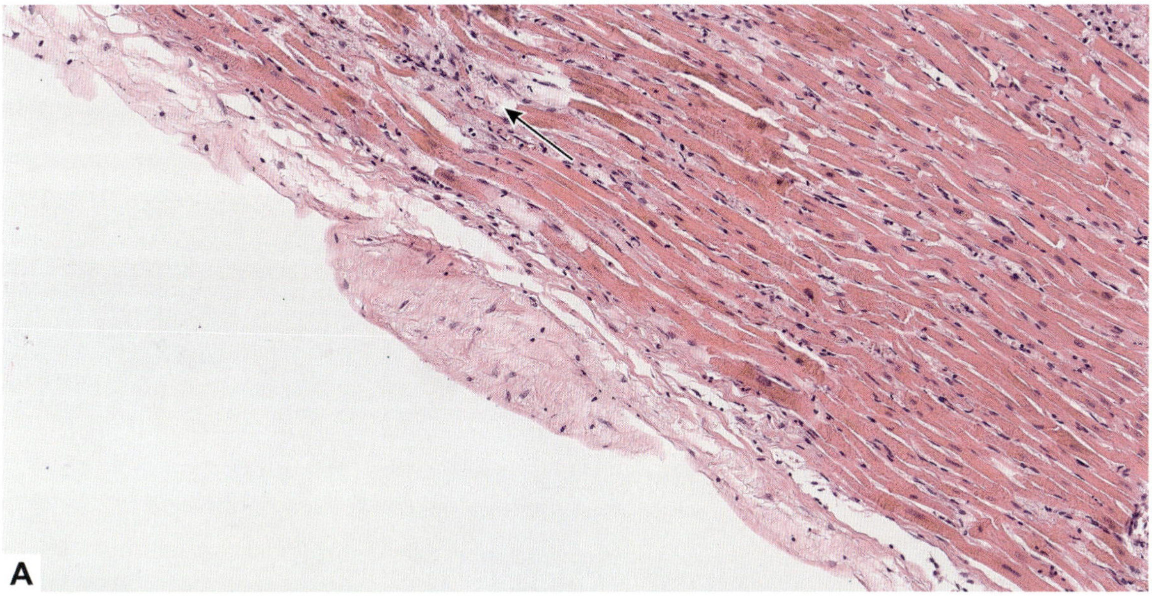

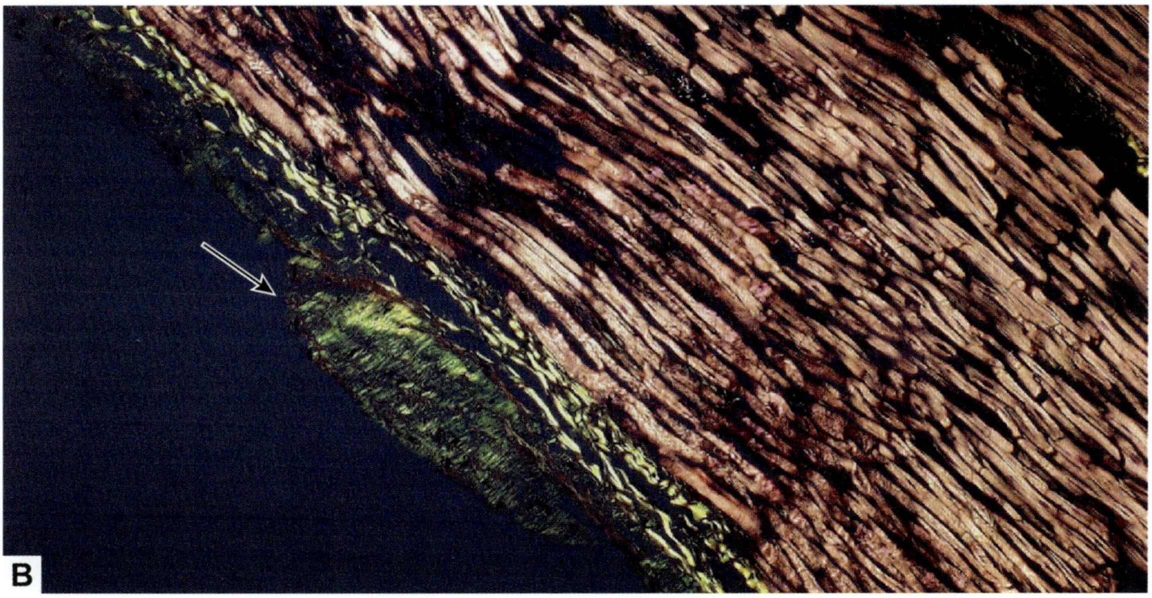

Fig. 1b2 Heart – Sequelae after pericarditis: Case 66 (48y m, case report p. 103)
A: Pericardial scar with marked thickening of the pericardium in places. In addition, subtle features of myocarditis with loose interstitial scarring (arrow). HE 100x.
B: Scarred, thickened pericardium with amyloid-like characteristics. Already in routine staining in polarised light birefringent, greenish shimmering aspect (arrow). HE 100x.

Continued on the next page.

c) Deposits

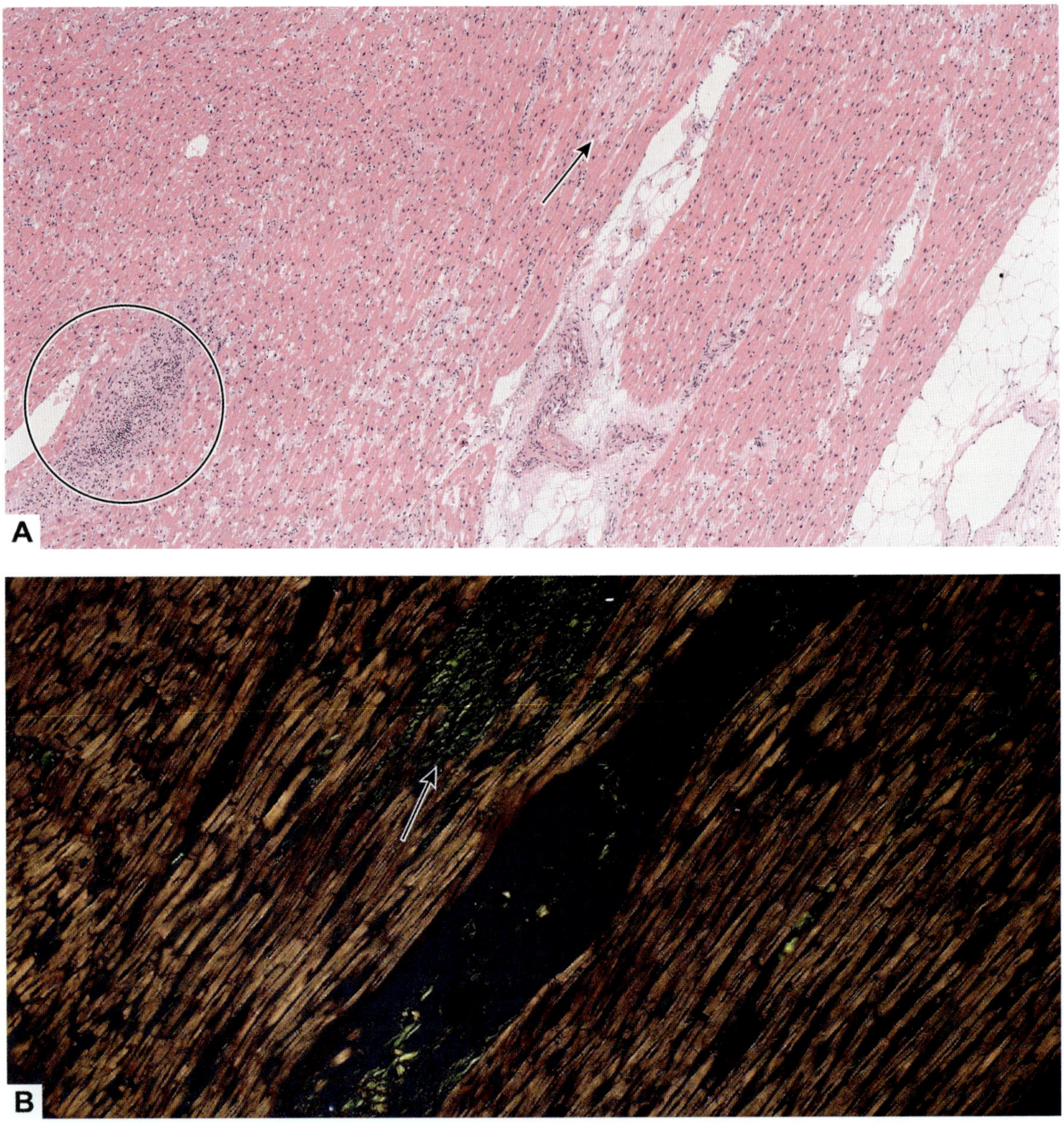

Fig. 1c1 Heart – Amyloid-like deposits, myocarditis: Continued case 66 (48y m, case report p. 103)
A: Focal lymphocytic infiltrate of the myocardium (circle) and fine-spotted scarring (arrow). HE 50x.
B: Fine-spotted perivascular and interstitial scarring (arrow) with perivascular and interstitial greenish birefringent, amyloid-like deposits already seen in routine staining in polarised light. HE 100x.

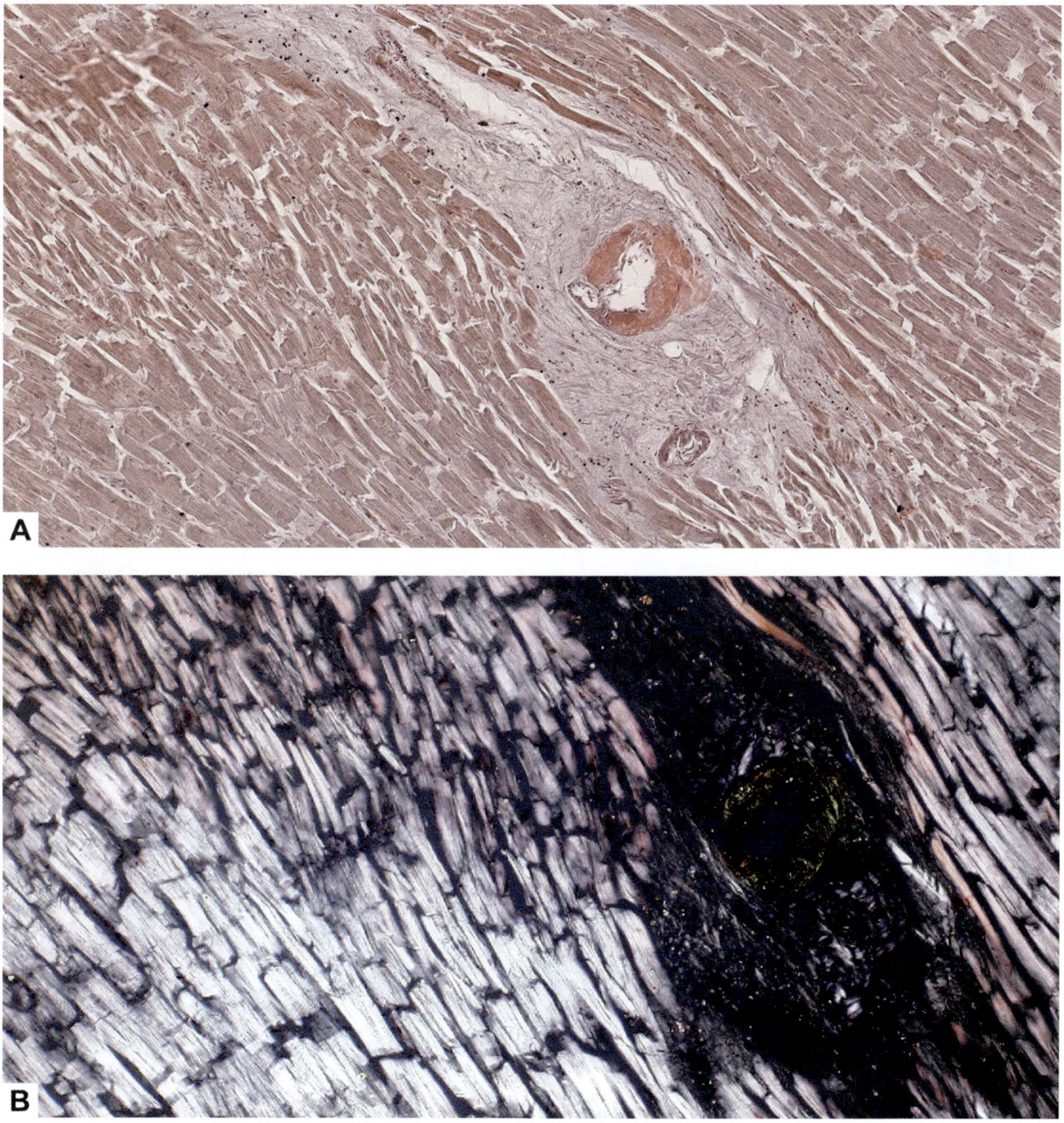

Fig. 1c2 Heart – Amyloid-like deposits: Case 104 (73y f, case report p. 113)
A: Circular amyloid deposit in a smaller intramural vessel with a more intense red colour in the special stain Congo red. Congo red 150x.
B: In polarised light, greenish shimmering, birefringent material, matching amyloid. Congo red 150x.

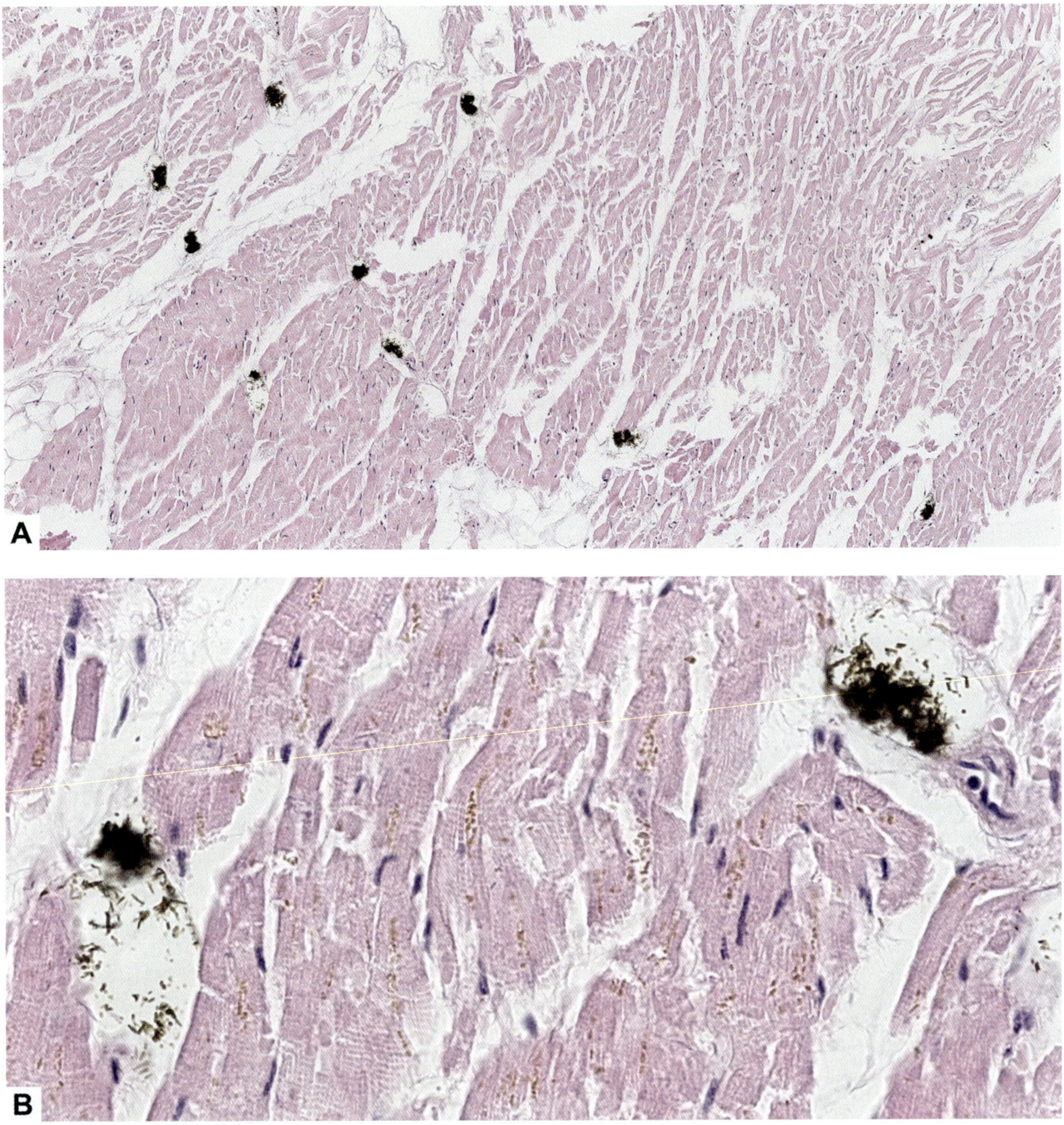

Fig. 1c3 Heart – Crystalline deposits of uncertain origin: Case 12 (81y f, case report p. 80)
A: Patchy deposit of black appearing crystalline material. HE 100x.
B: Roundish configured deposits of partly rod-shaped, partly needle-shaped material, which is not compatible with formalin pigment. HE 500x.

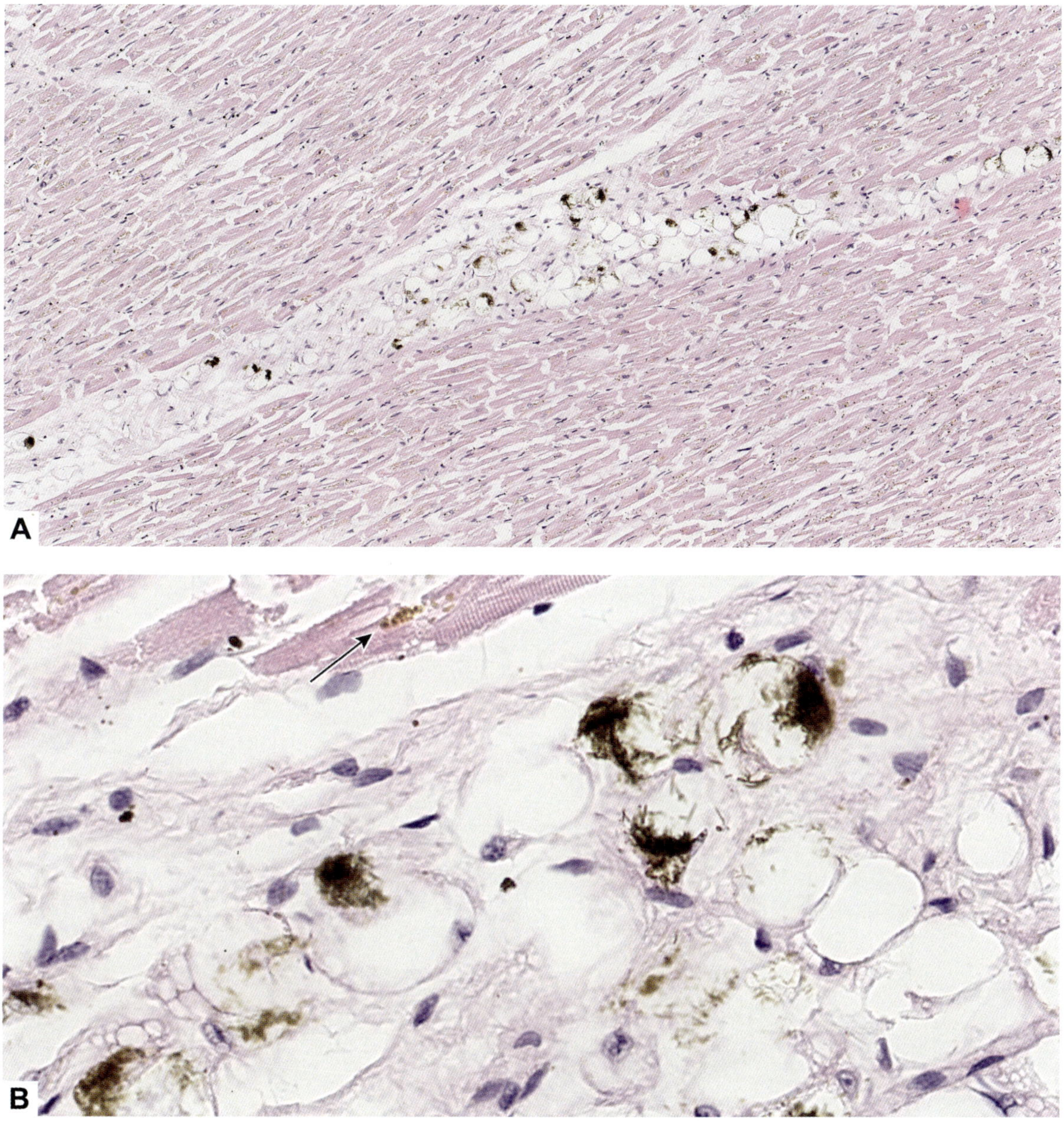

Fig. 1c4 Heart – Crystalline deposits of uncertain origin: Case 1 (82y f, case report p. 71)
A: Material of uncertain origin apparently lying in the fatty tissue with a black-dark brown aspect. HE 100x.
B: Often needle-like deposits arranged in circular structures. For comparison, focal common lipofuscin deposit (arrow). HE 550x.

d) Vascular changes

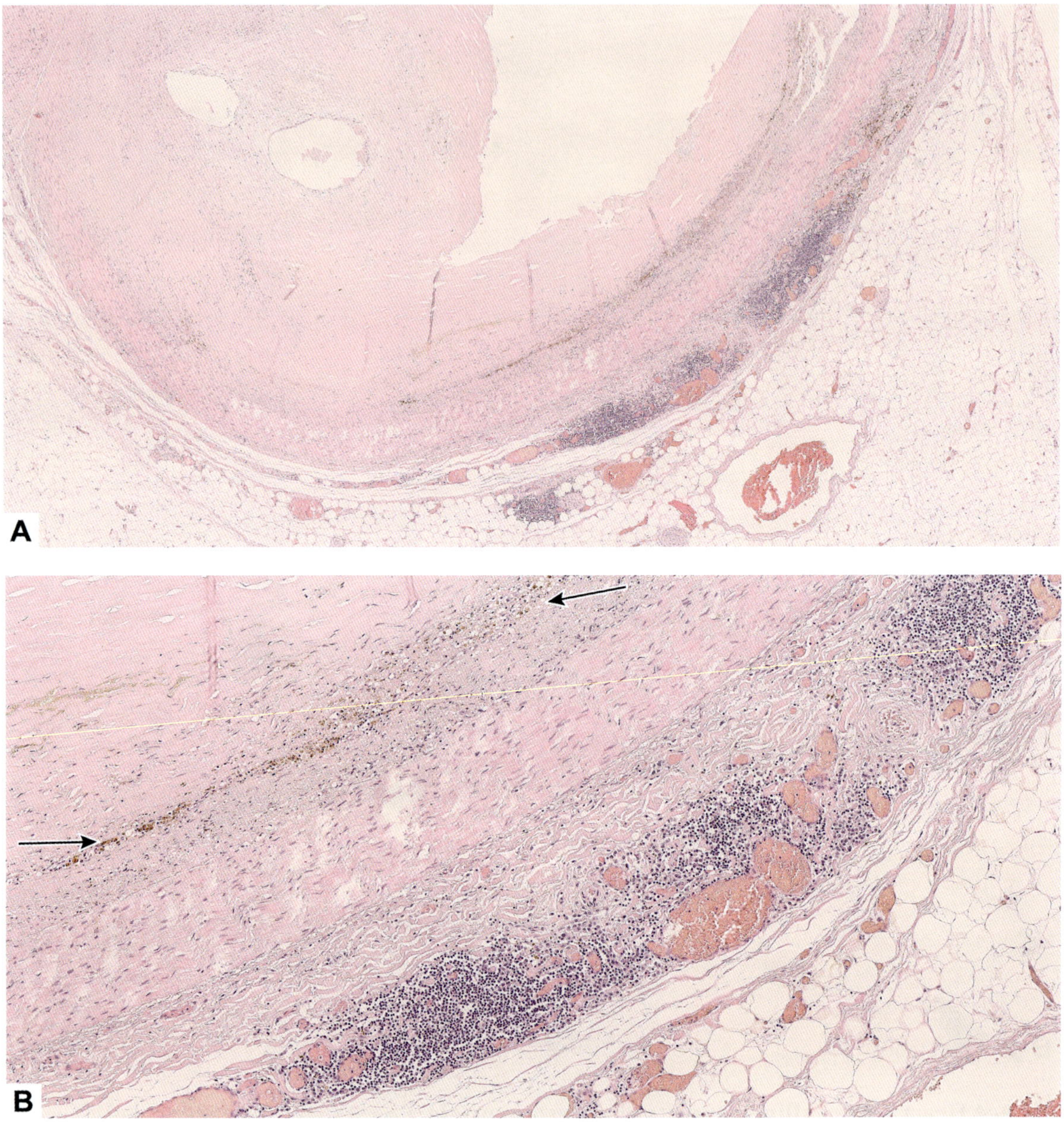

Fig. 1d1 Heart – Vascular changes: Case 49 (56y f, case report p. 97)
A: Atherosclerotic pre-damaged coronary artery with pronounced lumen-stenosing intimal fibrosis with recanalisation. Perivascular band-shaped lymphocytic infiltrate in places. HE 30x.
B: Intimal fibrosis with sparse lymphocytic infiltrate and haemosiderophages as features of older bleeding (arrows), adventitia with dense lymphocytic infiltrate, frequently around dilated blood-filled vasa vasorum. HE 80x.

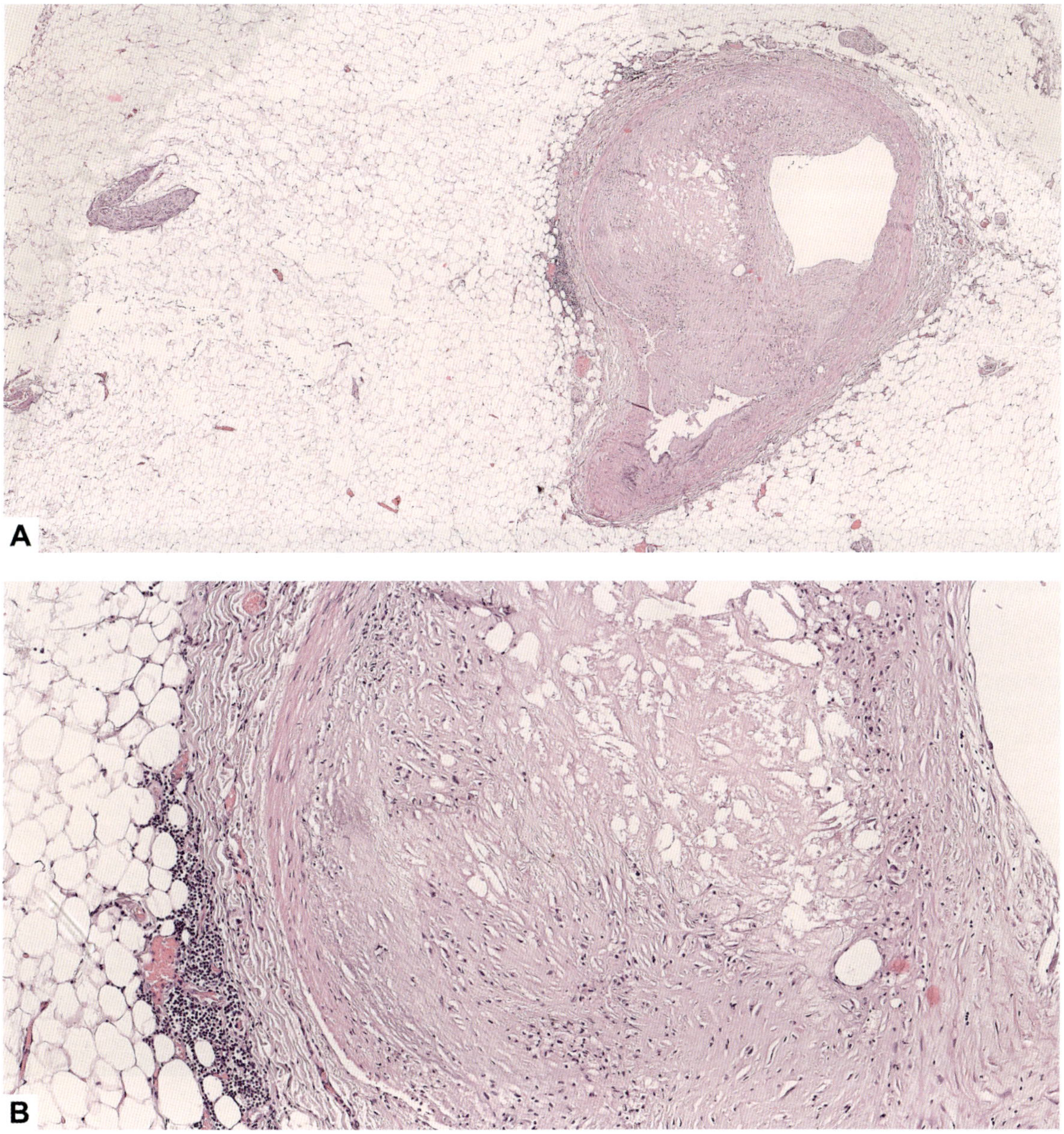

Fig. 1d2 Heart – Vascular changes: Case 58 (93y f, case report p. 99)
A: Coronary artery with pronounced lumen-stenosing intimal fibrosis consistent with atherosclerotic pre-damage. HE 30x.
B: Disintegrating plaque and mild infiltration by lymphocytes and macrophages as well as perivascular lymphocytic infiltration. HE 100x.

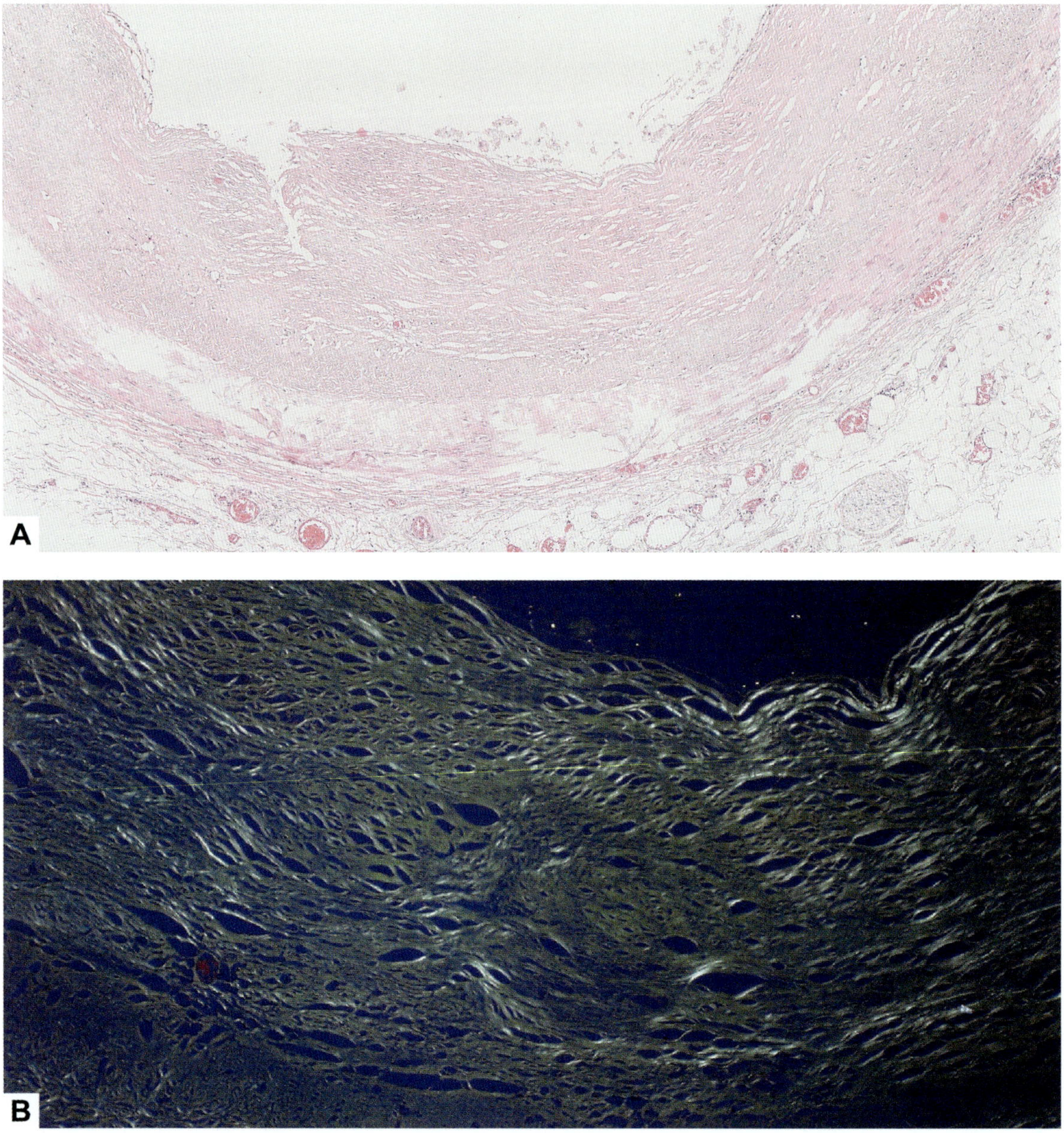

Fig. 1d3 Heart – Vascular changes: Case 83 (72y m, case report p. 109)
A: Intimal fibrosis with conspicuous oedematous loosening. HE 100x.
B: Intimal fibrosis with clearly visible oedematous loosening in polarised light. HE 150x.

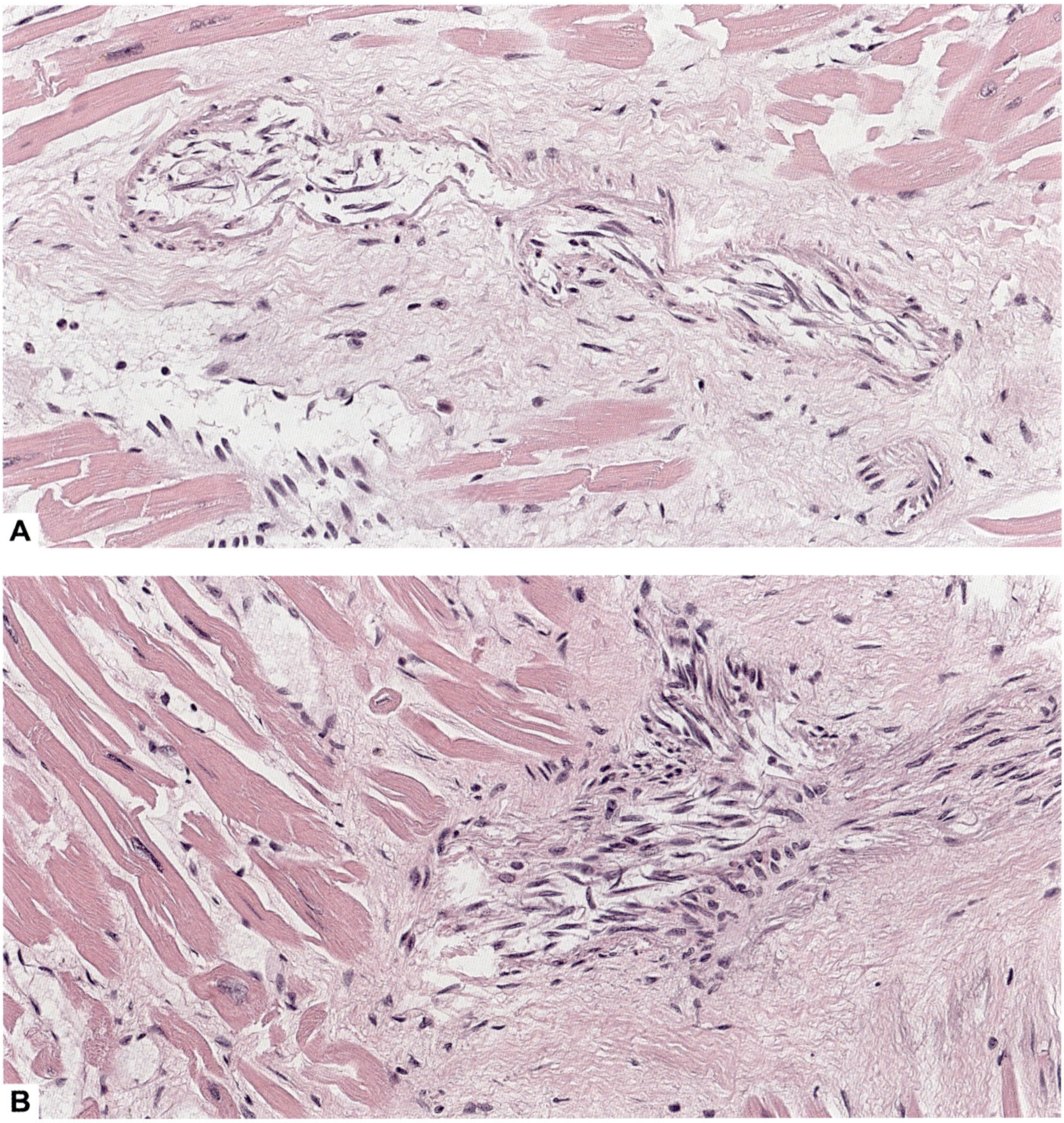

Fig. 1d4 Heart – Vascular changes: Case 20 (59y f, case report p. 85)
A+B: Smaller intramural vessels with exfoliated, reactively enlarged endothelia in the lumen and single lymphocytes consistent with endothelialitis. Mild perivascular and interstitial fibrosis. HE 200x.

e) Ischaemic phenomena

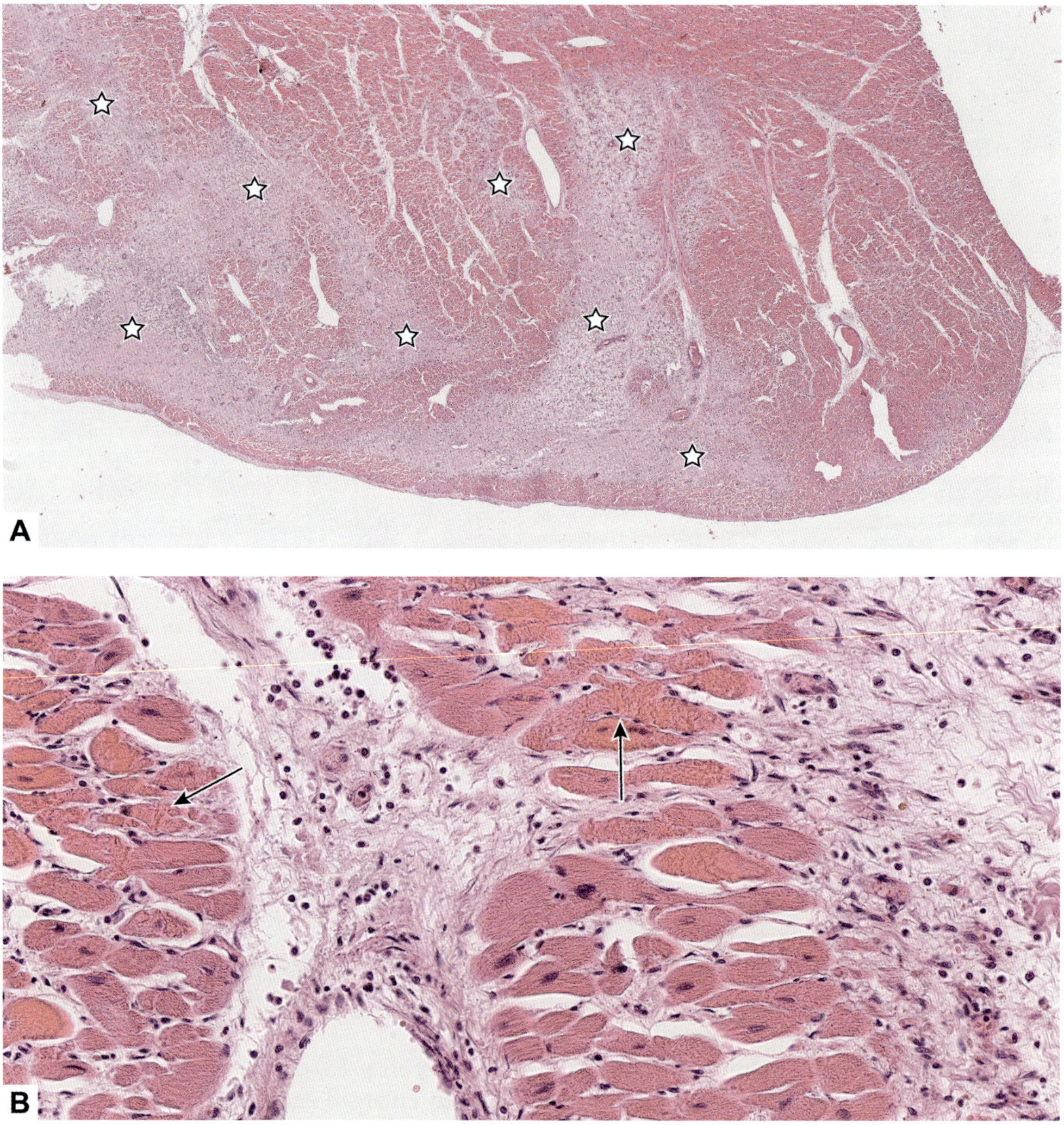

Fig. 1e Heart – Ischaemic phenomena: Case 72 (24y m, case report p. 104)
A: Band-like confluent granulation tissue foci (asterisks) and features of acute myocardial infarction with more strongly eosinophilic stained myocardium in the border area of the scars. HE 20x.
B: Loose granulation tissue with infiltration by predominantly neutrophil granulocytes, acute myocardial necrosis, partly with indicated contraction band necrosis (arrows) and more strongly eosinophilic stained cardiomyocytes. HE 200x.

2. Spleen

a) Vascular changes

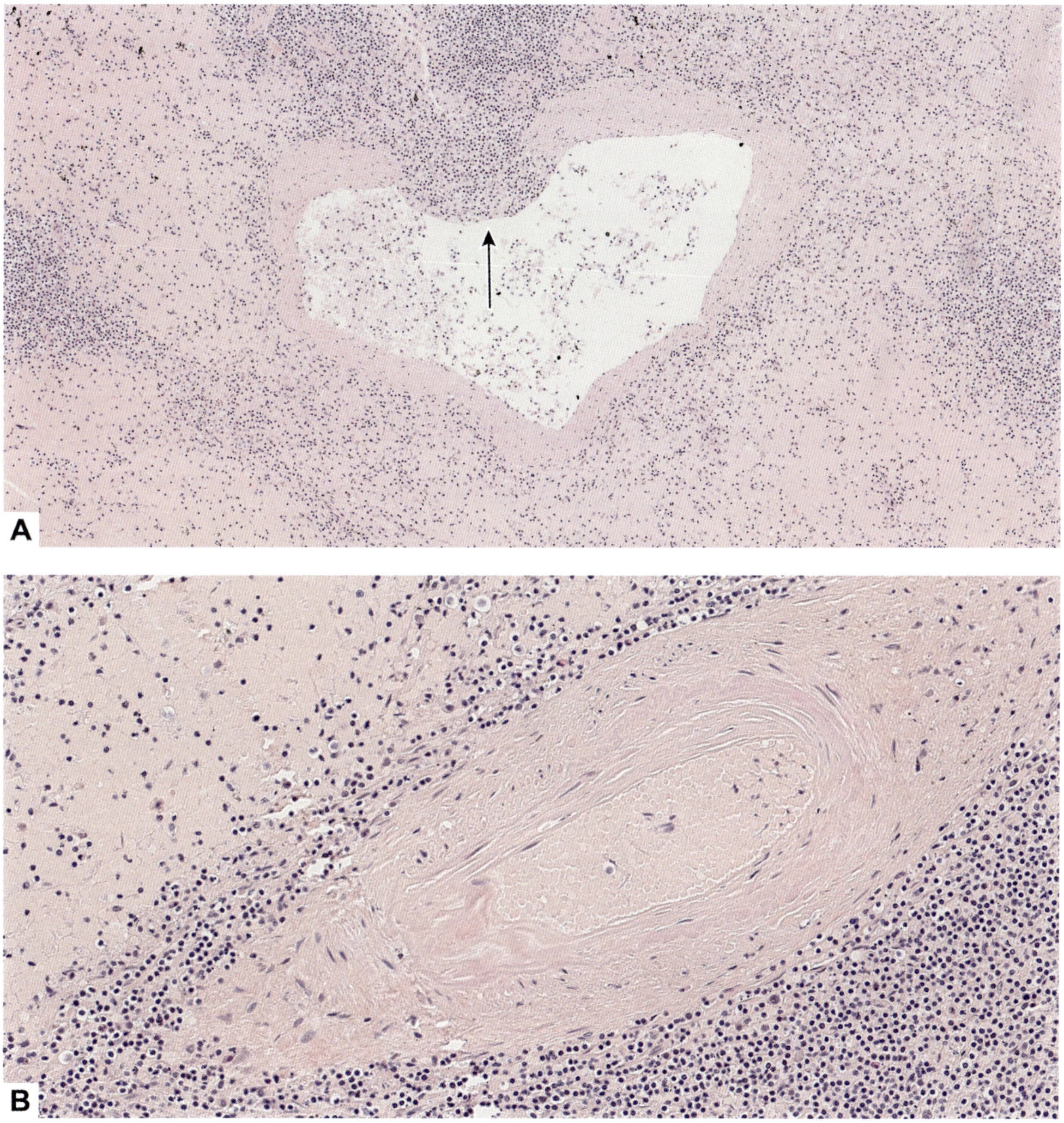

Fig. 2a1 Spleen – Vascular changes: Case 17 (83y f, case report p. 82)
A: Architectural distortion of the wall of a medium calibre vessel with follicular invasion into the vessel lumen (arrow), an abnormality detectable at several sites in this spleen. HE 70x.
B: Onion-skin-like phenomenon of the vessel wall of an artery (also seen in several other arterial vessels of the spleen). HE 200x.

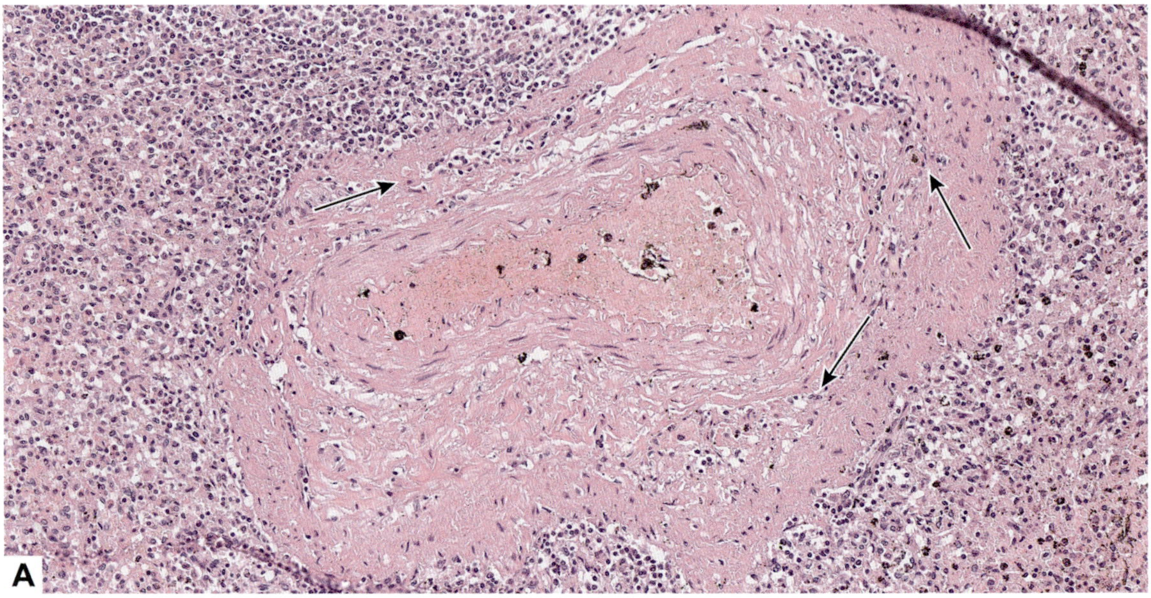

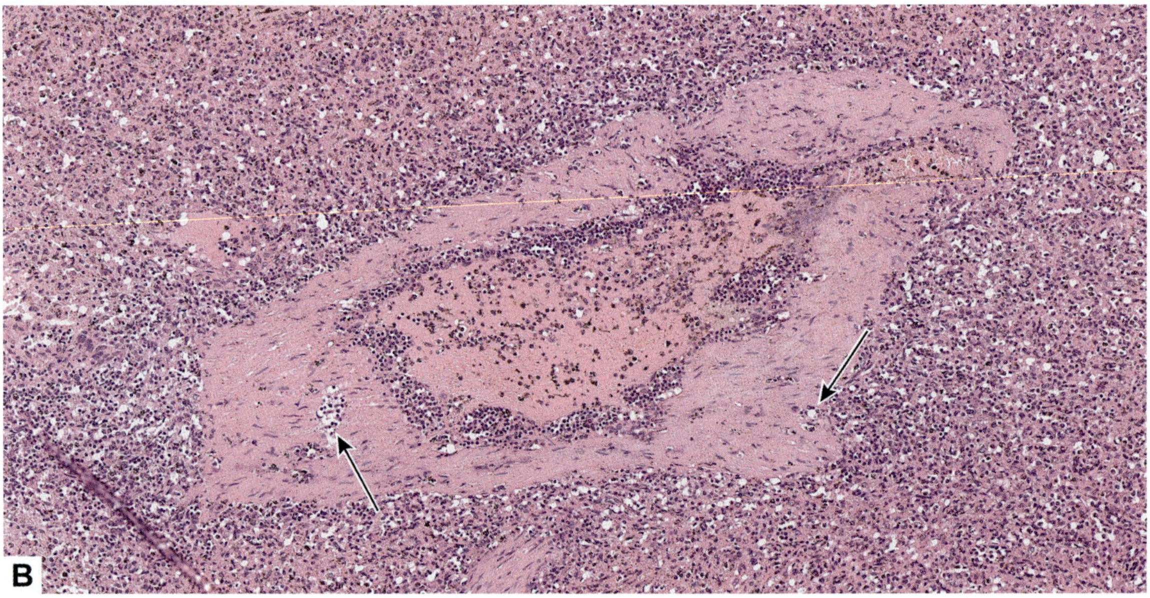

Fig. 2a2 Spleen – Vascular changes: Case 18 (29y m, case report p. 83)
A: Medium-sized arterial vessel with oedematous loosened wall layers and the image of the so-called onion-skin pattern as well as inflammatory lymphocytic infiltrates in the outer wall layers (arrows) consistent with vasculitis. HE 160x.
B: Medium-sized arterial vessel with the picture of vasculitis, massive circular infiltration by lymphocytes close to the lumen; individual lymphocytes can also be found in deeper wall layers (arrows). HE 100x.

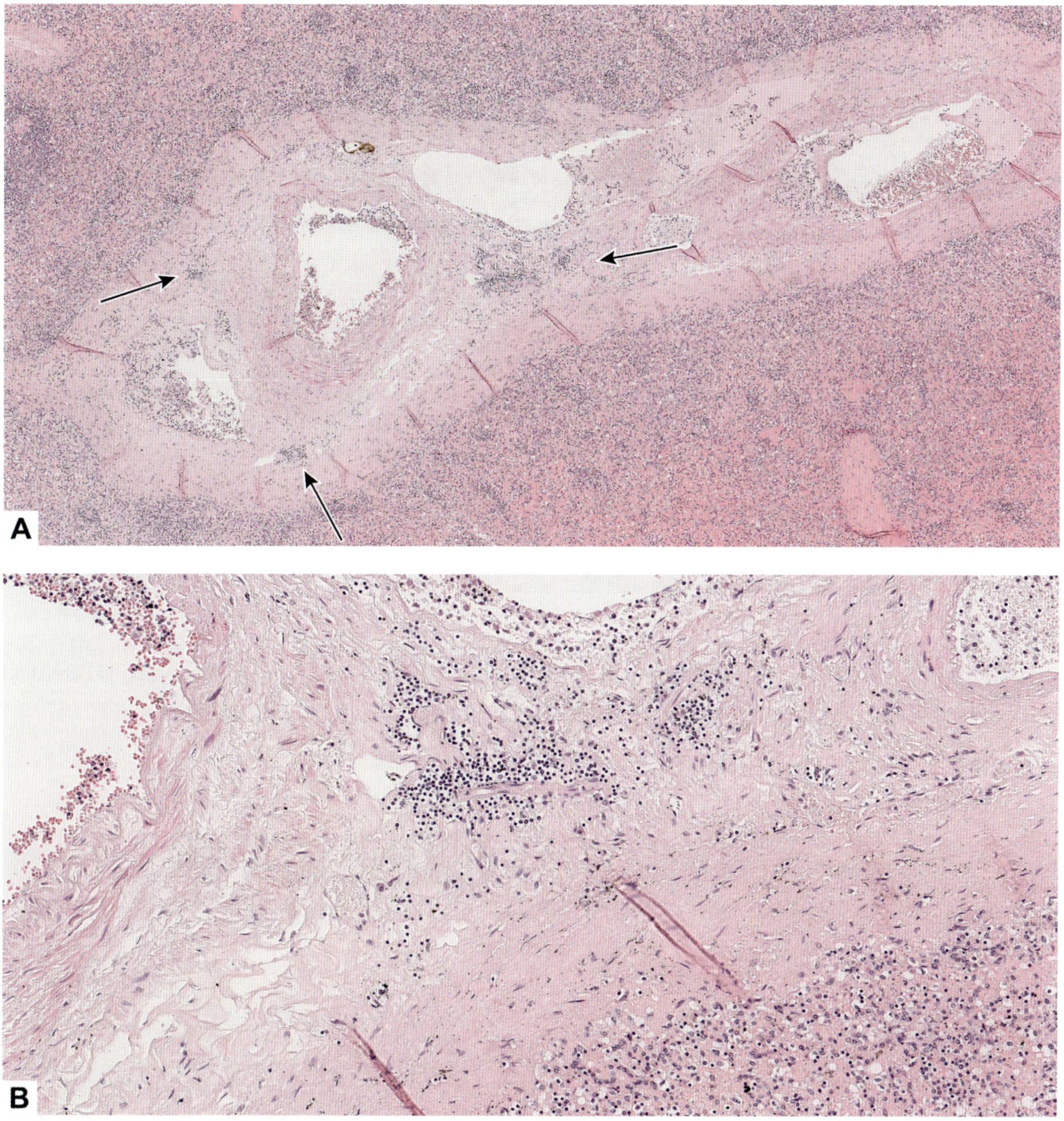

Fig. 2a3 Spleen – Vascular changes: Case 2 (71y m, case report p. 73)
A: Larger calibre arterial vessel with loosened wall structure and focal infiltration by lymphocytes (arrows). HE 40x.
B: Relatively dense lymphocytic infiltration of the inner vessel wall layers in places. HE 130x.

b) Deposits

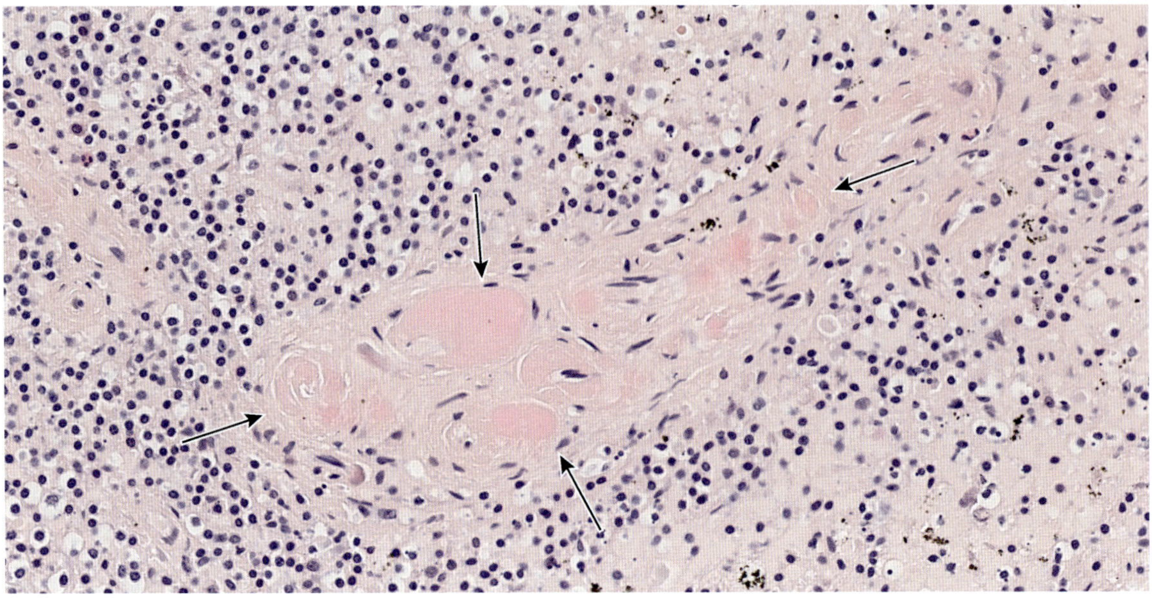

Fig. 2b Spleen – Deposits: Case 17 (83y f, case report p. 82)
Partly circumferential, homogeneous eosinophilic deposits in the wall of capillary vessels (arrows) consistent with amyloid-like deposits. HE 300x.

3. Liver

a) Inflammatory changes

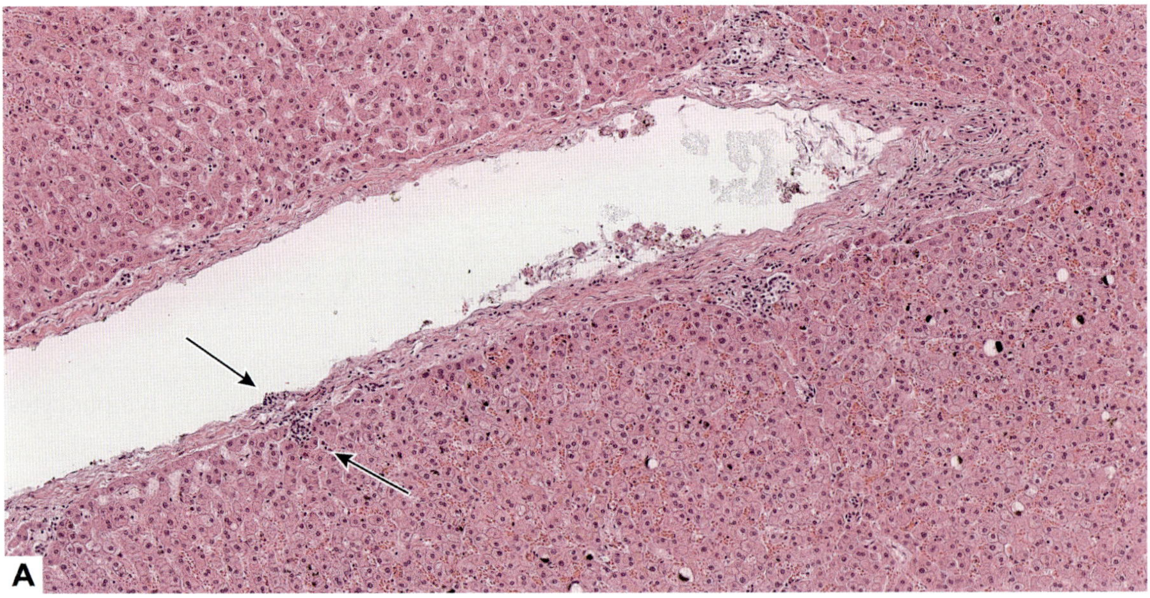

Fig. 3a Liver – Inflammatory changes: Case 30 (39y m, case report p. 90)
A: Dilated vein in the portal tract with focal inflammatory infiltrate (arrows). HE 100x.

Continued on the next page.

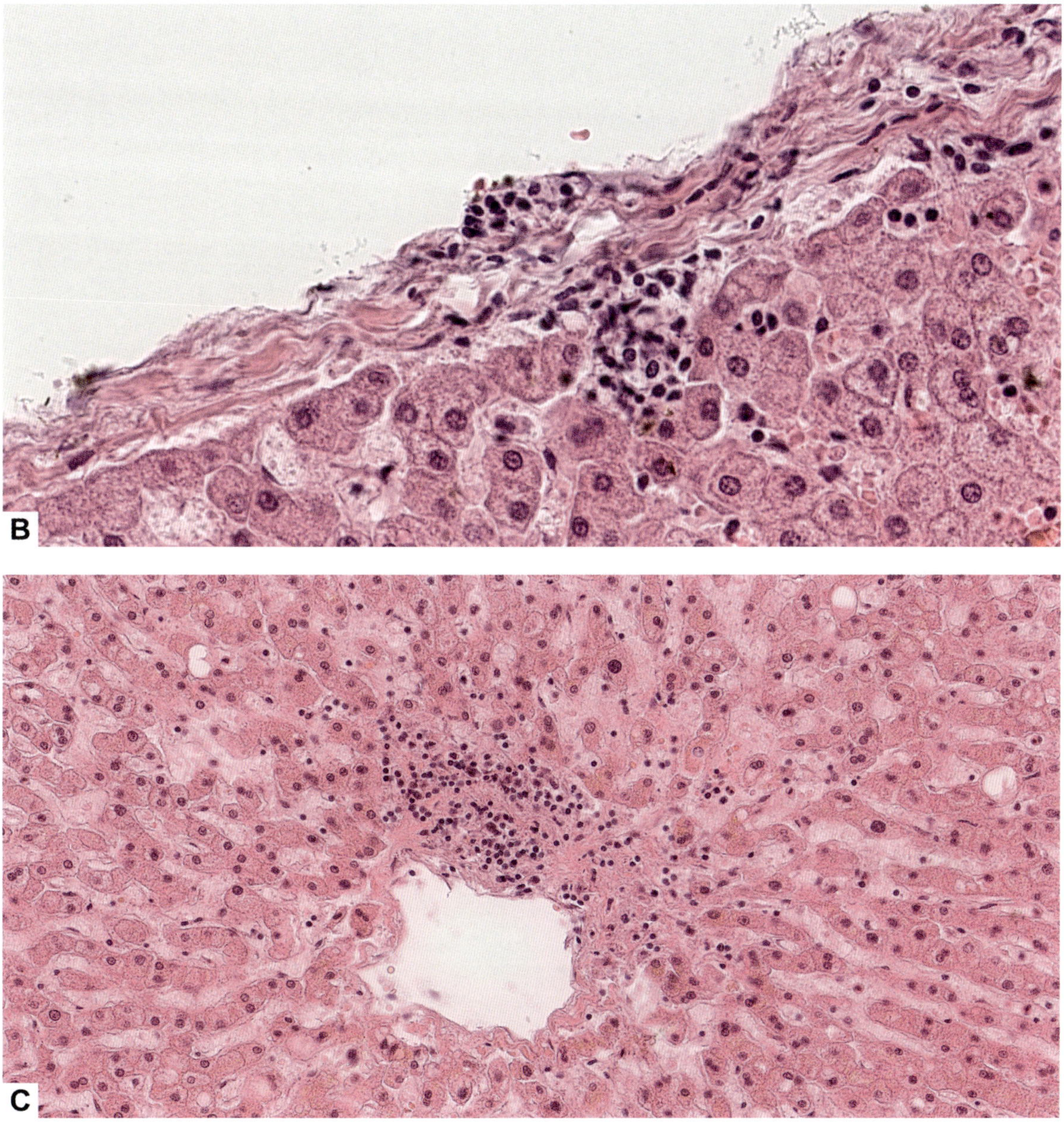

Fig. 3a Liver – Inflammatory changes: Continued case 30 (39y m, case report p. 90)
B: Portal vein with minimal inflammatory infiltrate with mild interface hepatitis. HE 500x.
C: Central vein with inflammatory infiltrate spreading to the hepatic lobule. HE 200x.

b) Deposits

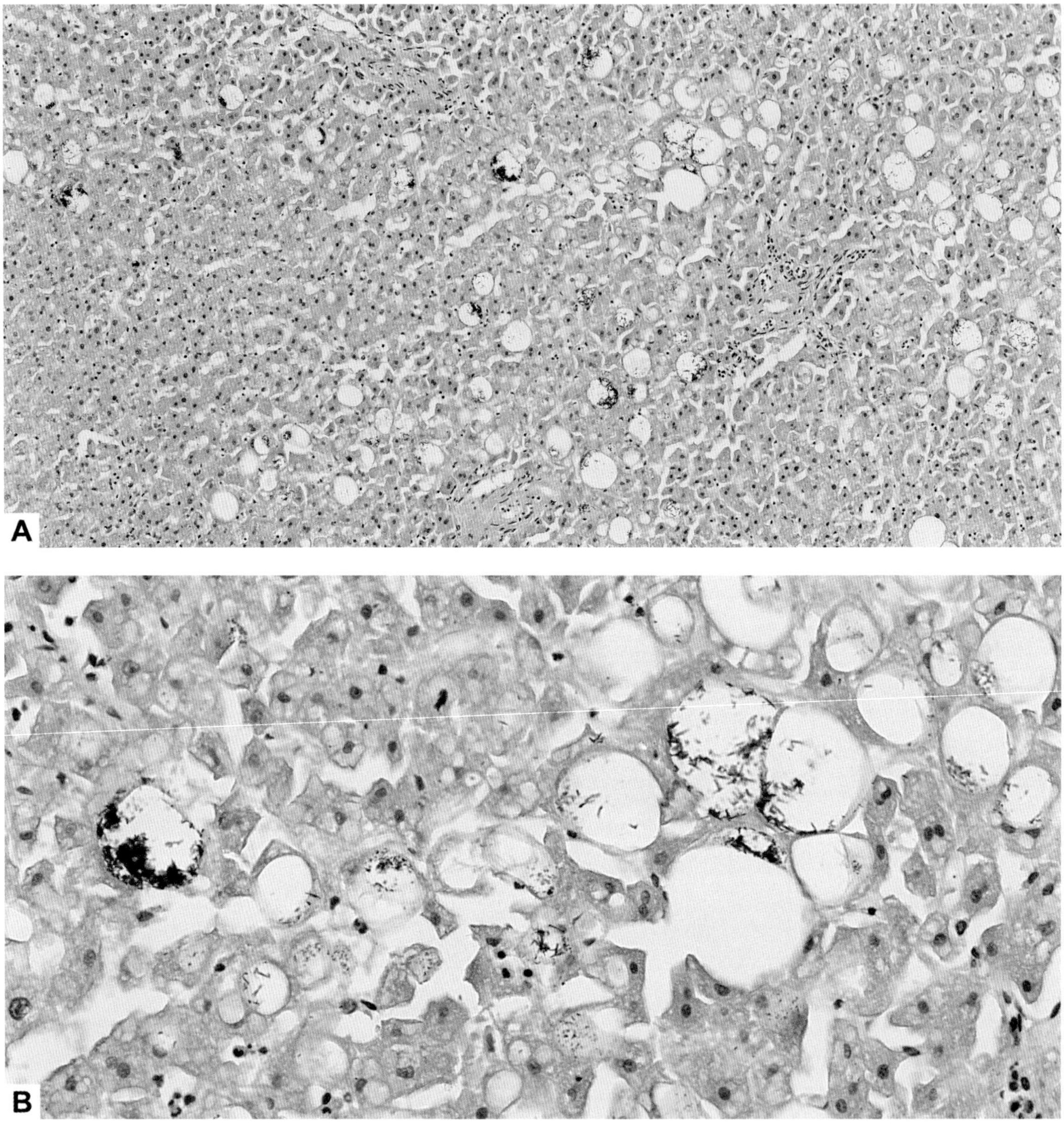

Fig. 3b1 Liver – Deposits: Case 18 (29y m, case report p. 83)
A: Moderate steatosis with accumulation of black appearing crystalloide material of uncertain origin in the fat vacuoles. HE 100x.
B: Macro- and microvesicular steatosis and needle-shaped or crystalloide material of uncertain origin, mostly seen in the large fat vacuoles. HE 300x.

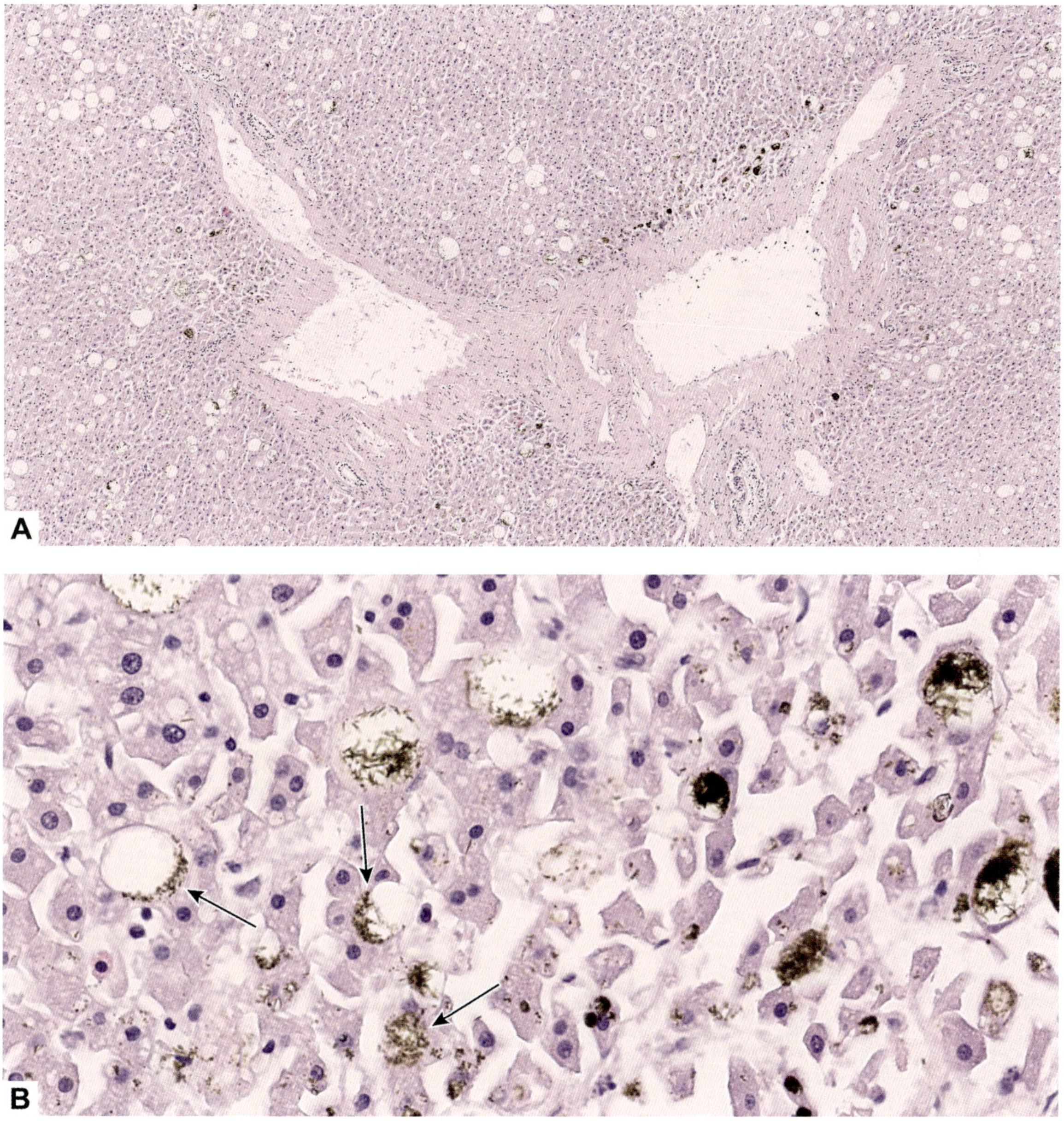

Fig. 3b2 Liver – Deposits: Case 13 (63y m, case report p. 81)
A: Fatty degeneration of hepatocytes with periportal accentuated brown-black appearing crystalloide material of uncertain origin. HE 50x.
B: Macro- and microvesicular steatosis with brown-black crystalloide material of uncertain origin in the fat vacuoles, often in a needle-like configuration, but sometimes also present in shorter fragments (arrows). HE 400x.

4. Brain

a) Inflammatory changes

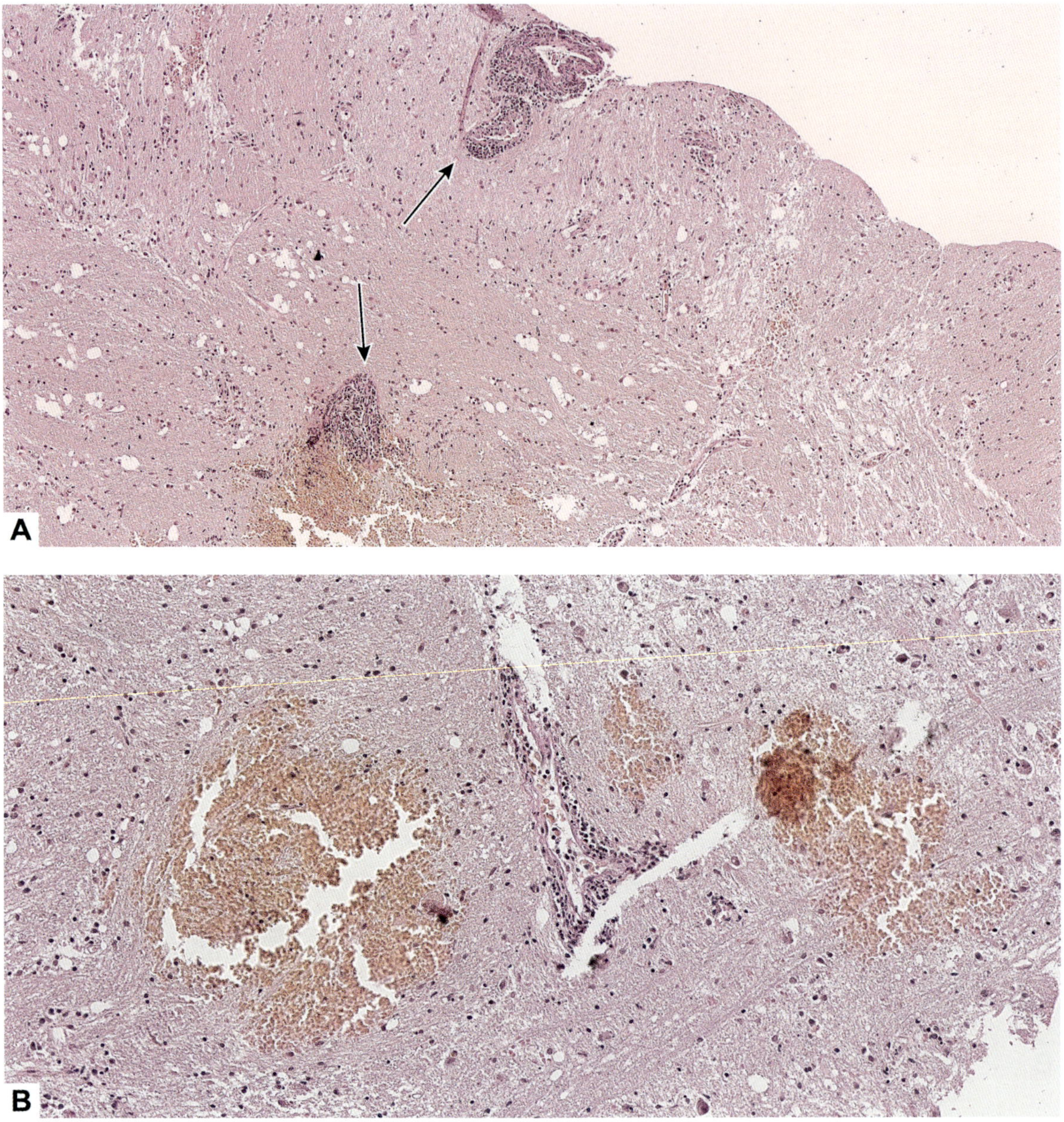

Fig. 4a Brain – Inflammatory changes, haemorrhages, infarction: Case 120B (63y f, case report p. 129)
A: Clear inflammatory component with dense lymphocyte infiltrates in the area of the vessels (arrows), patchy acute haemorrhage, acute cerebral infarction with interstitial oedema of the brain substance and early microglial and macrophagocytic reaction. Crush artefacts due to biopsy trauma, especially in the vascular area. HE 100x.
B: Vessel with lymphocytic infiltration, patchy, acute intracerebral haemorrhages and infarction with oedema and slightly increased intracerebral cellularity. HE 150x.

b) Haemorrhages

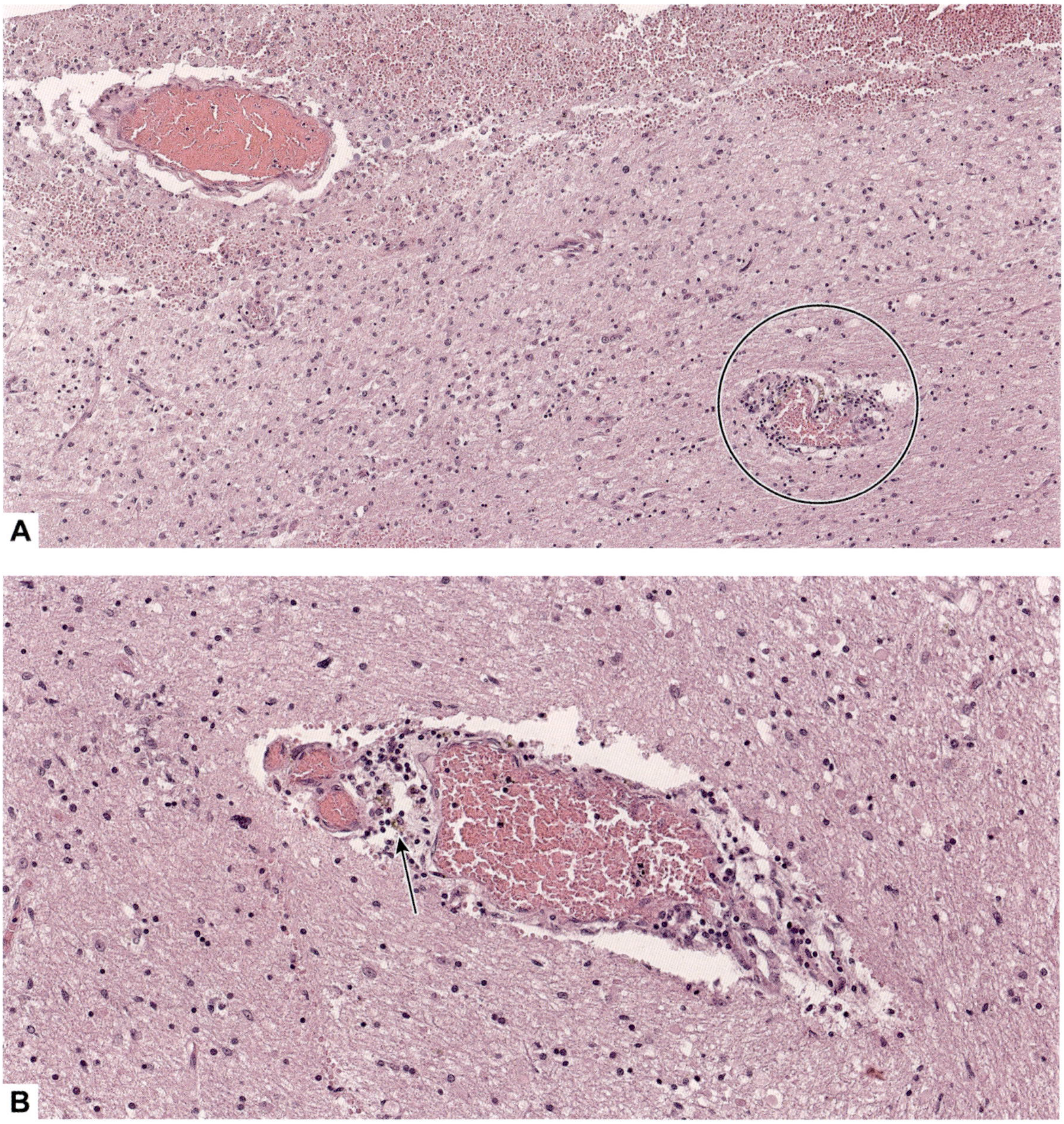

Fig. 4b Brain – Haemorrhages, inflammatory changes, infarction: Case 60 (72y f, case report p. 100)
A: Partially dilated blood-filled vessels, one with surrounding lymphocytic infiltrate (circle); patchy, fresh haemorrhages and relatively acute cerebral infarction with microglial and histiocytic reaction. HE 100x.
B: Another dilated vessel with surrounding lymphocytic infiltrate and individual haemosiderophages (arrow) as a feature of older haemorrhages. HE 150x

c) Infarction

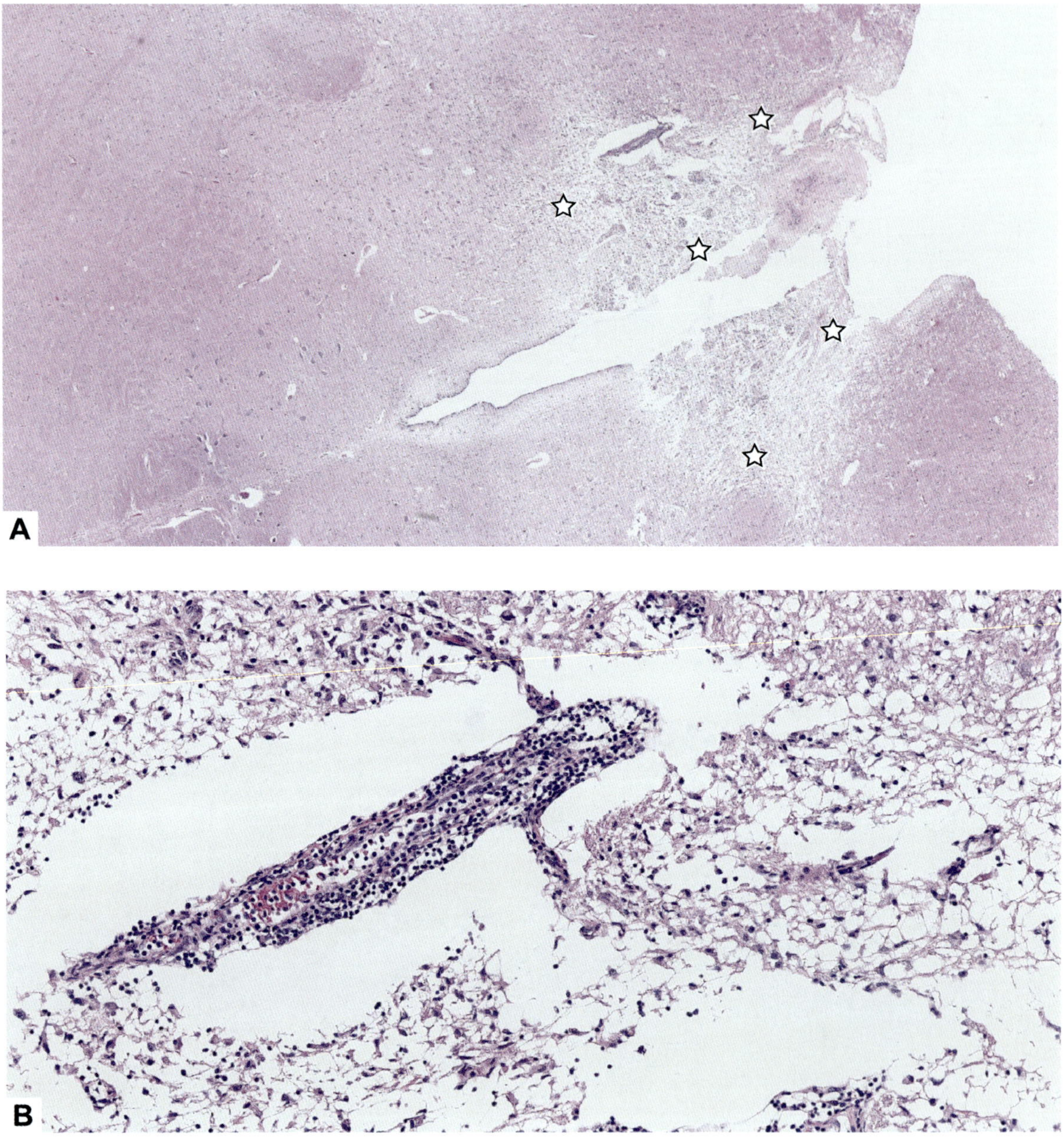

Fig. 4c Brain – Infarction, inflammatory changes: External case (61y m, case report p. 125)
A: Vasculitis with surrounding cerebral infarction (asterisks) in the medulla oblongata. HE 20x.
B: Oedematous widened vessel wall with dense lymphocytic infiltrate, which partially spreads to the brain tissue. Surrounding tissue with marked oedema. HE 150x.

5. Lung

a) Inflammatory changes

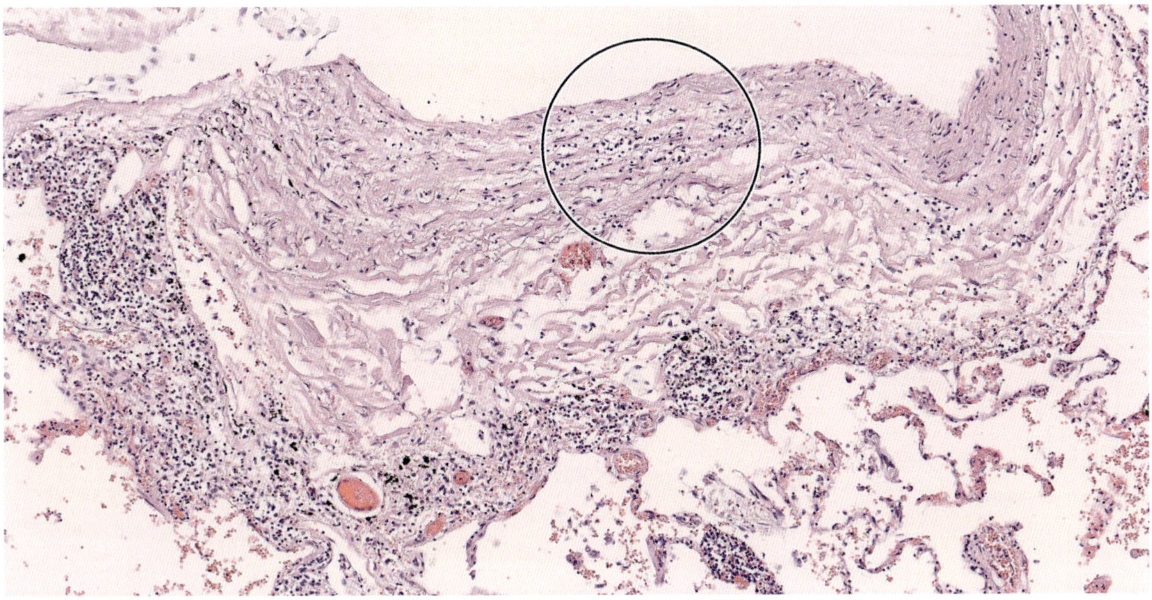

Fig. 5a1 Lung – Inflammatory changes: Case 13 (63y m, case report p. 81)
Large calibre blood vessel with pronounced perivascular lymphocytic infiltrate and loose lymphocytic infiltration of the vessel wall (circle). Patchy black pigment, consistent with black carbon pigment. HE 100x.

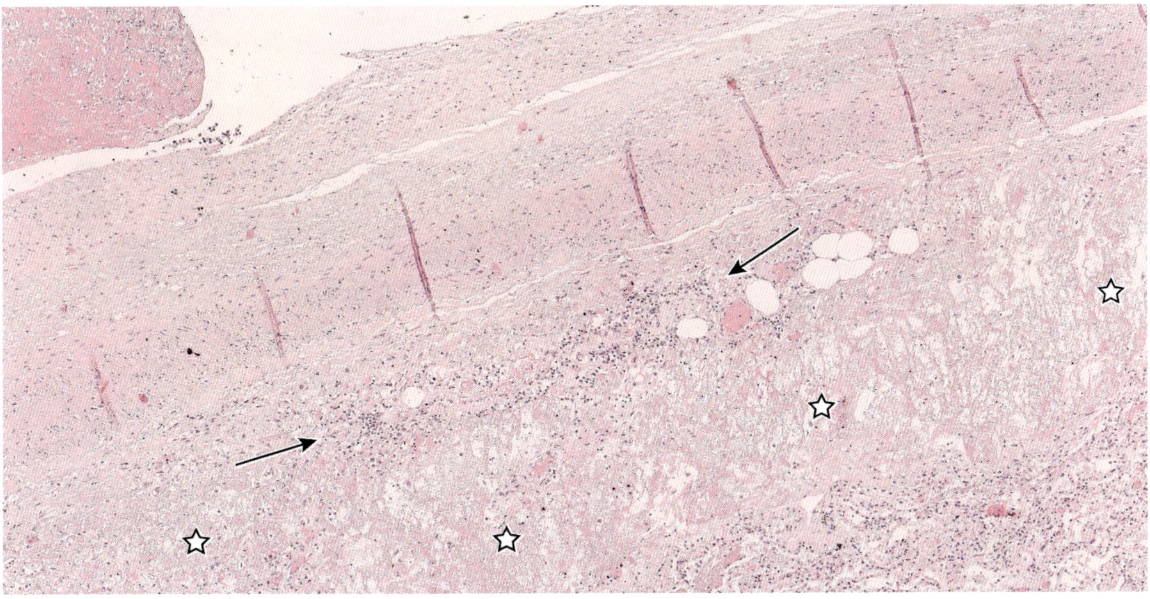

Fig. 5a2 Lung – Inflammatory changes, thrombus: Case 21 (85y m, case report p. 87)
Pulmonary artery with acute thrombus in the vessel lumen (top left of image). Degeneration of media with architectual distortion of stratifite elastic fibres, mild perivascular lymphocytic infiltrate (arrows), conspicuous perivascular oedema (asterisks). HE 50x.

b) Thrombi

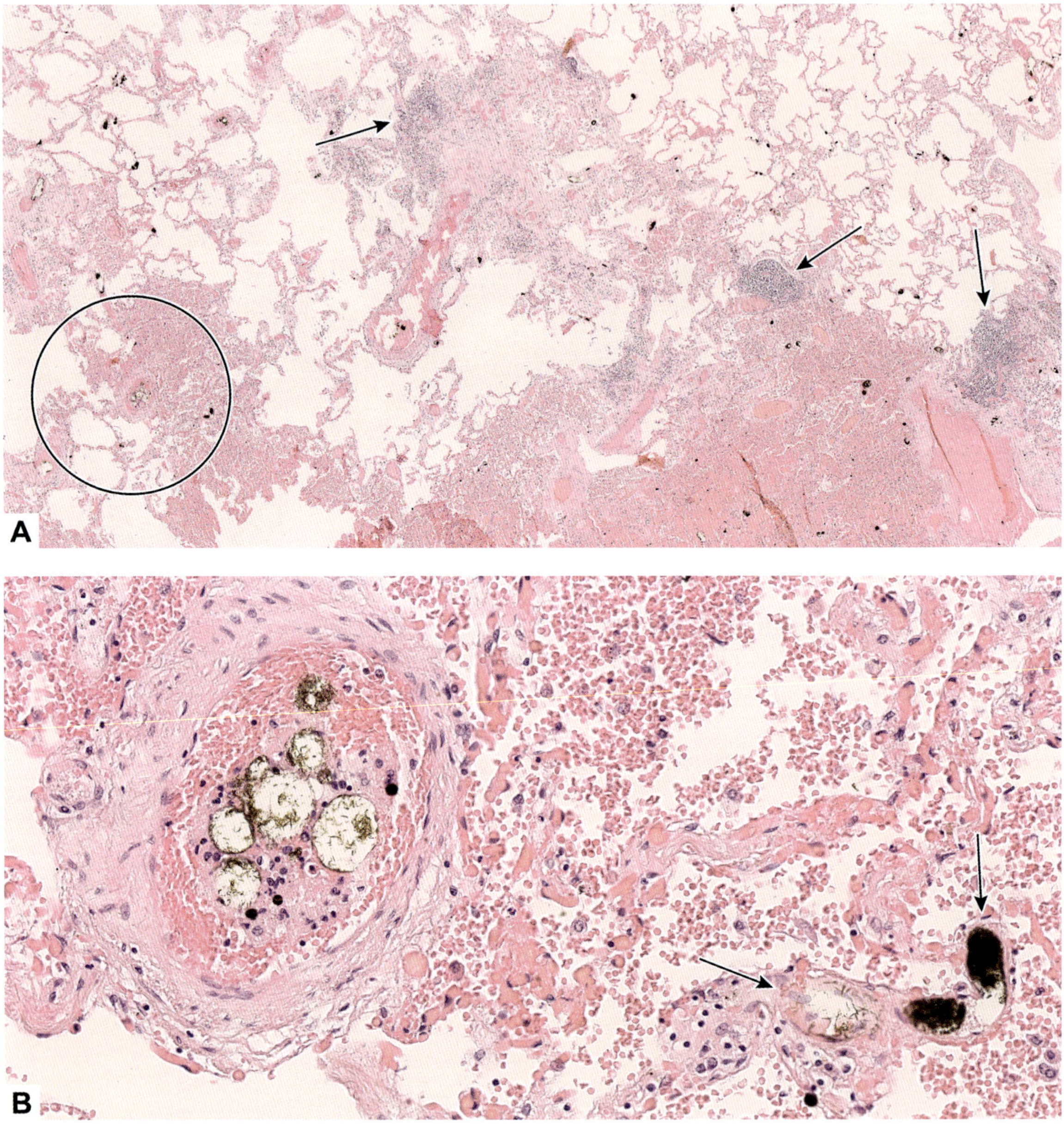

Fig. 5b Lung – Thrombi, haemorrhagic infarction, inflammatory changes, deposits:
Case 47 (51y m, case report p. 96)
A: In numerous capillary vessels and focally also in a medium calibre blood vessel (circle) black appearing crystalloide deposits of uncertain origin, picture of haemorrhagic infarction, patchy interstitial lymphocytic infiltrate (arrows). HE 20x.
B: In a medium calibre pulmonary artery, drop-like crystalloide material of uncertain origin, consisting of rod-shaped dark brown aggregates, consistent with a foreign body embolism. Also capillary vessels with similar material in the lumen (arrows). HE 200x.

c) Deposits

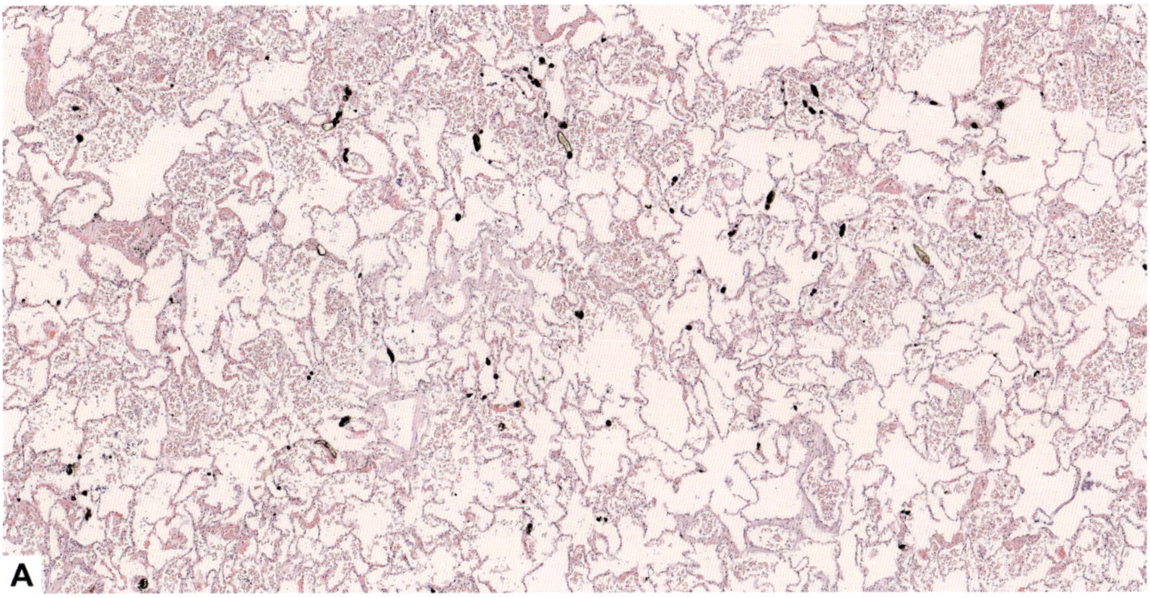

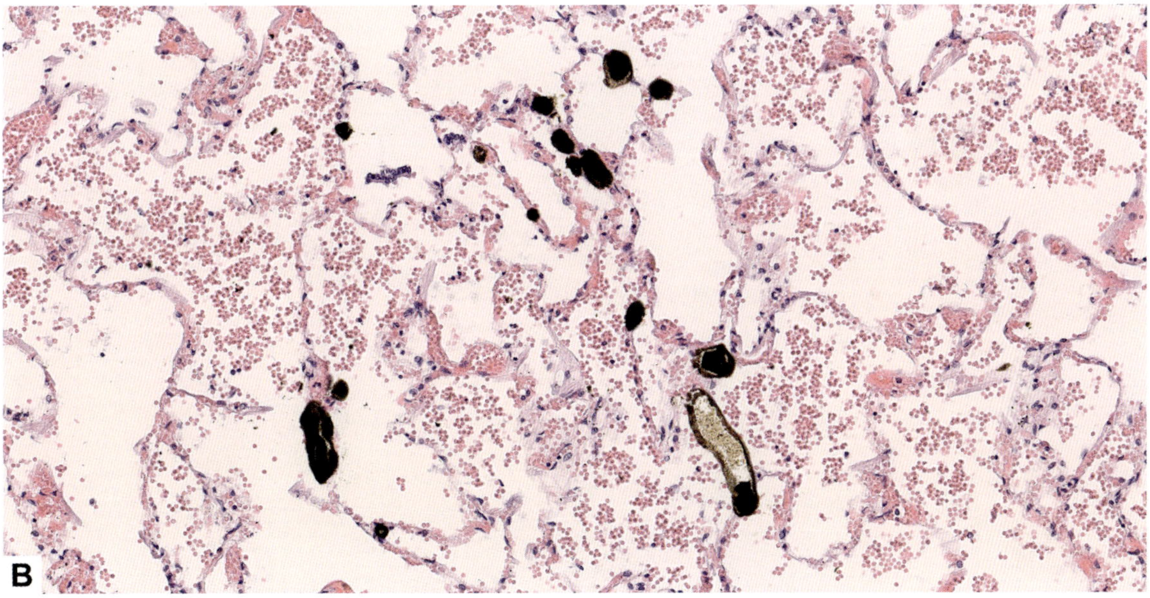

Fig. 5c1 Lung – Deposits: Case 13 (63y m, case report p. 81)
A: Crystalloide deposits of uncertain origin appearing black in numerous capillary vessels. Features of acute congestion. HE 20x.
B: In addition to hyperaemia, the black crystalloide material, primarily localised in capillary vessels, is conspicuous and fills some of the lumina completely. HE 150x.

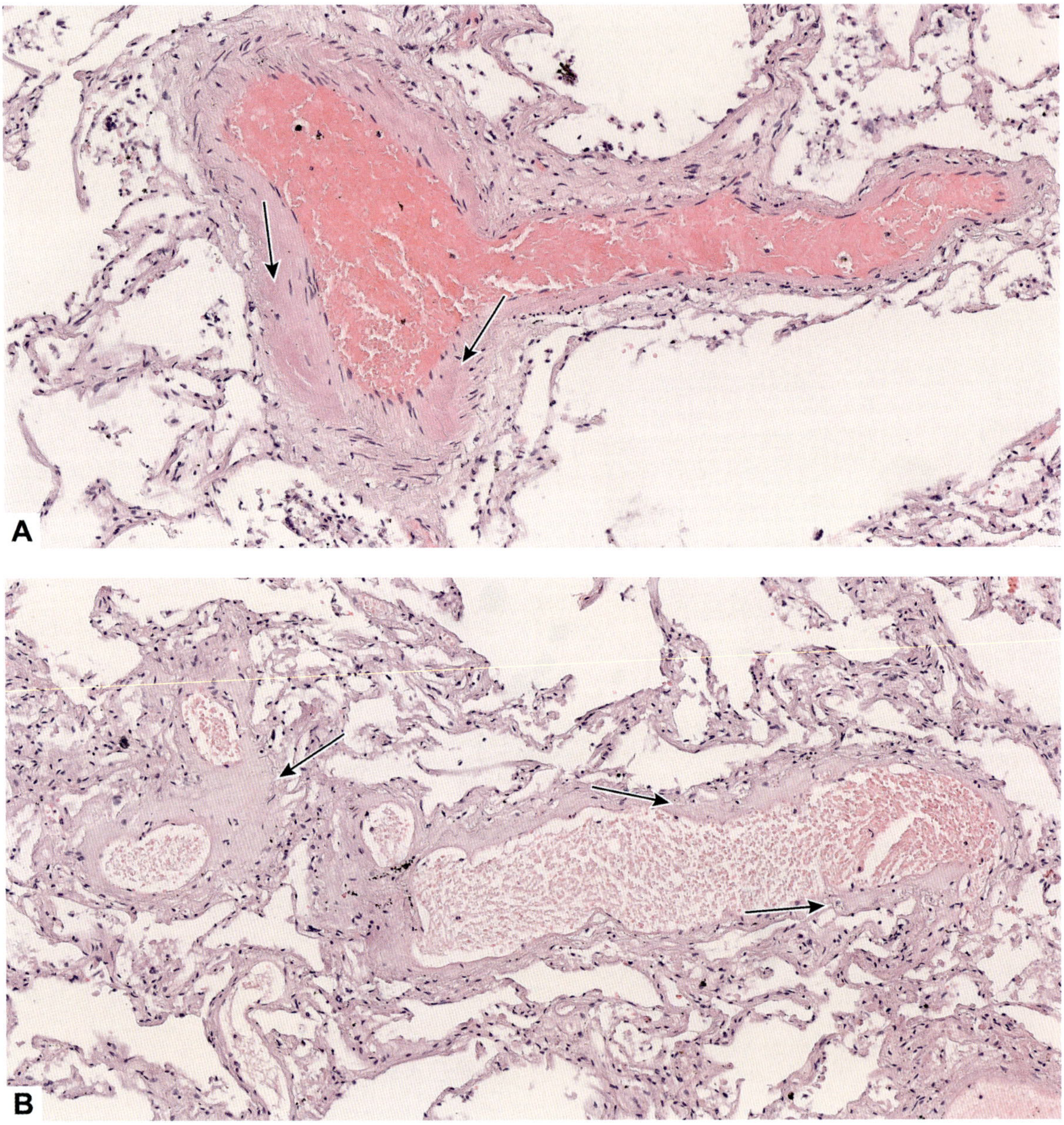

Fig. 5c2 Lung – Deposits: Case 3 (94y f, case report p. 74)
A+B: In numerous places in the wall of smaller blood vessels, indicated cushion-shaped thickening or circularly arranged deposits of homogeneous, in part strongly eosinophilic coloured material (arrows). HE 100x.

6. Thyroid gland

a) Inflammatory changes

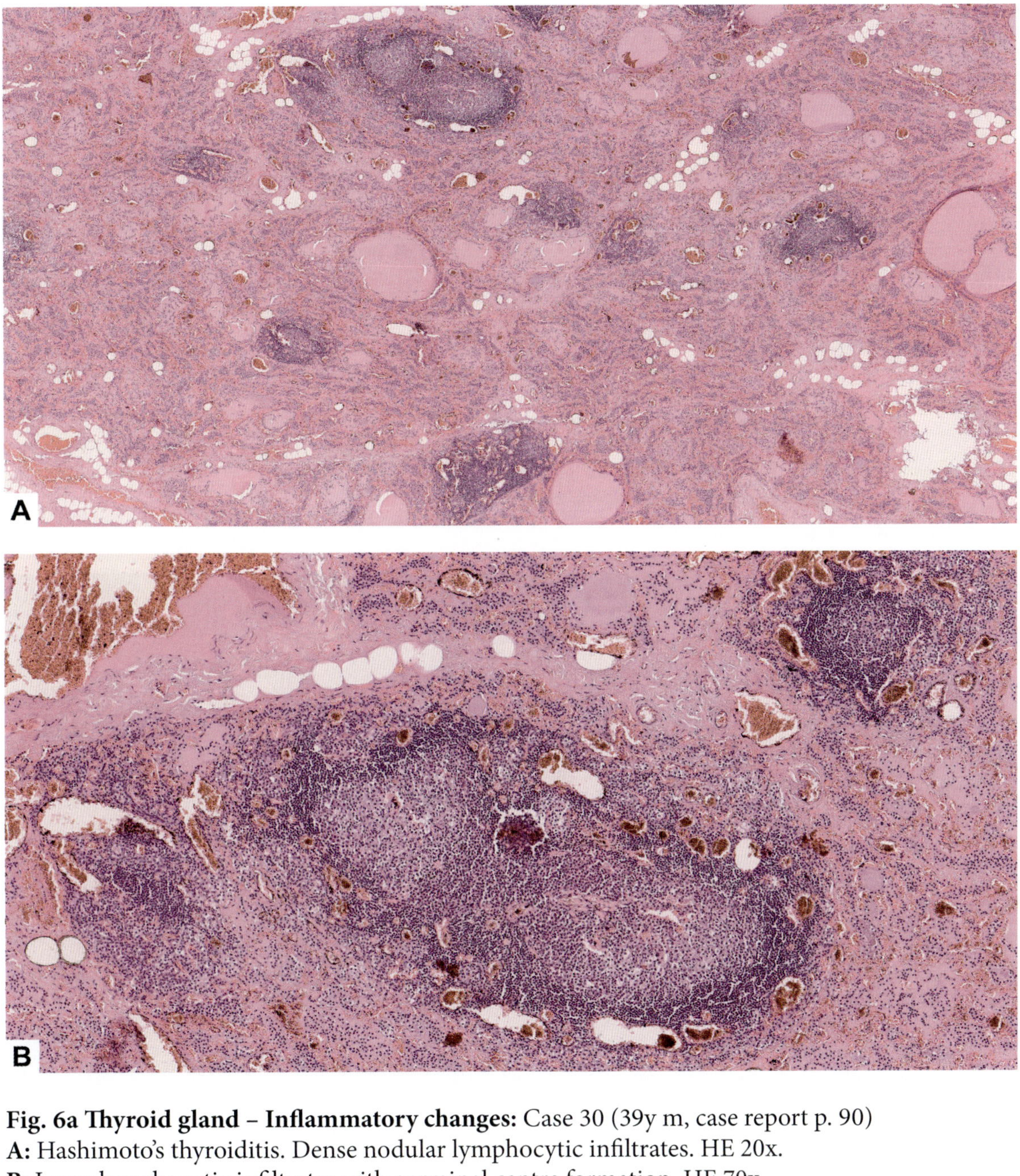

Fig. 6a Thyroid gland – Inflammatory changes: Case 30 (39y m, case report p. 90)
A: Hashimoto's thyroiditis. Dense nodular lymphocytic infiltrates. HE 20x.
B: Large lymphocytic infiltrates with germinal centre formation. HE 70x.

7. Adrenal gland

a) Deposits

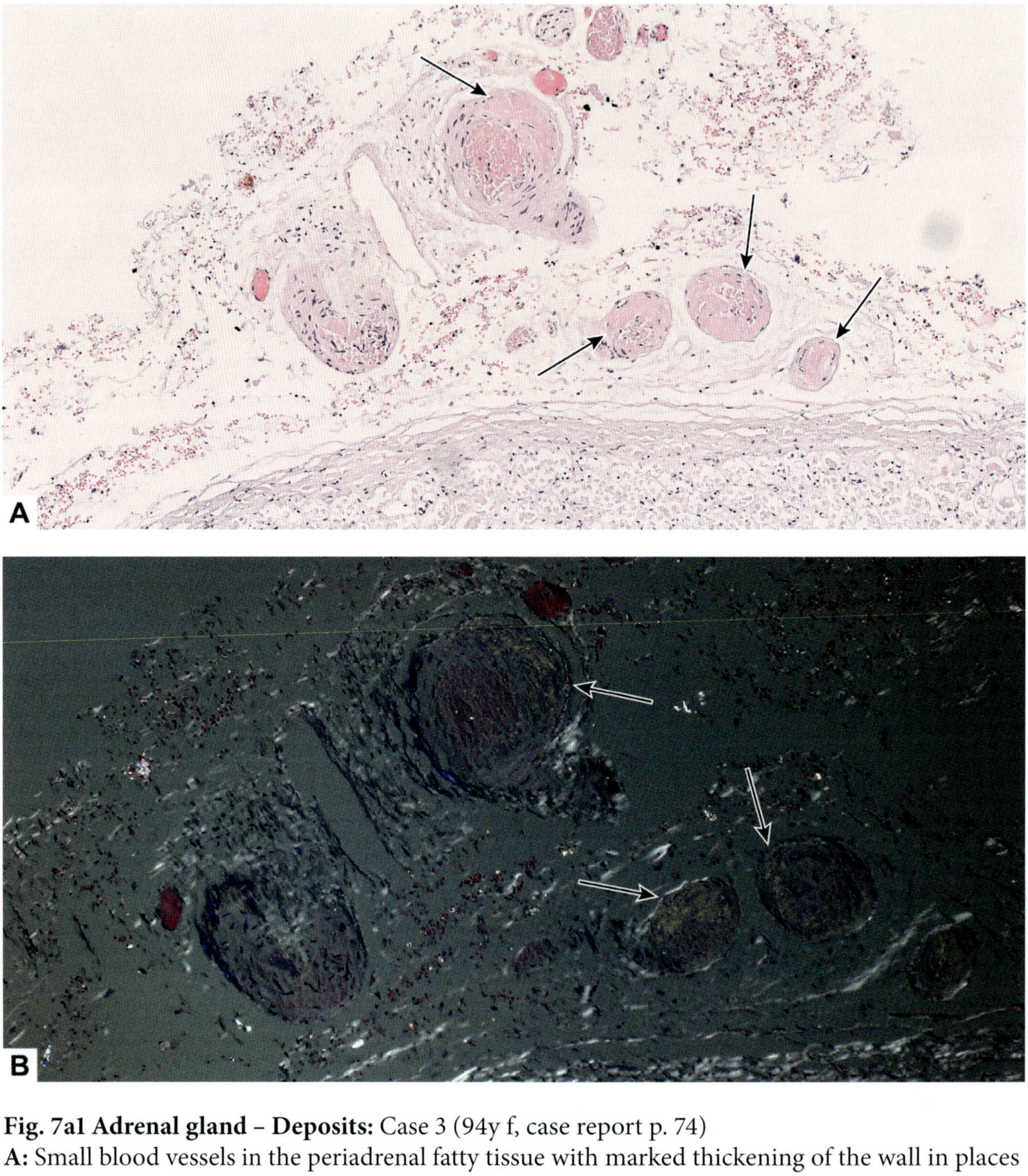

Fig. 7a1 Adrenal gland – Deposits: Case 3 (94y f, case report p. 74)
A: Small blood vessels in the periadrenal fatty tissue with marked thickening of the wall in places and homogeneous, strongly eosinophilic coloured deposits (arrows). HE 100x.
B: Readyly seen in routine staining in polarised light slightly greenish birefringent (arrows). HE 150x.

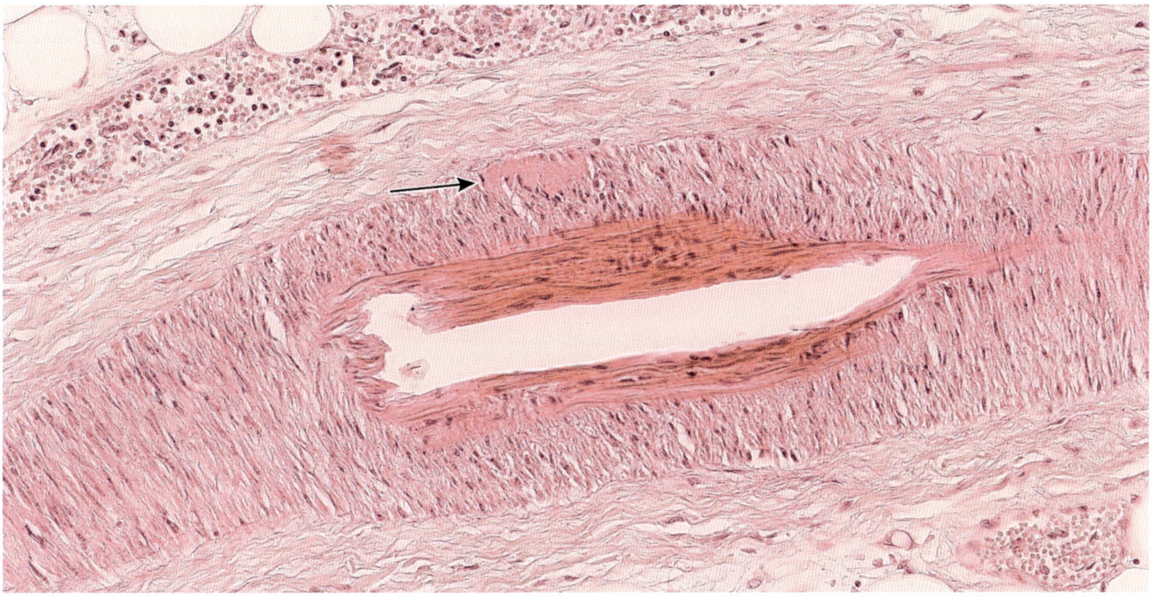

Fig. 7a2 Adrenal gland – Deposits: Case 9 (89y f, case report p. 78)
Larger arterial vessel in the periadrenal adipose tissue with focally very discreet deposition of homogeneous, more eosinophilic material (arrow), consistent with amyloid. HE 180x.

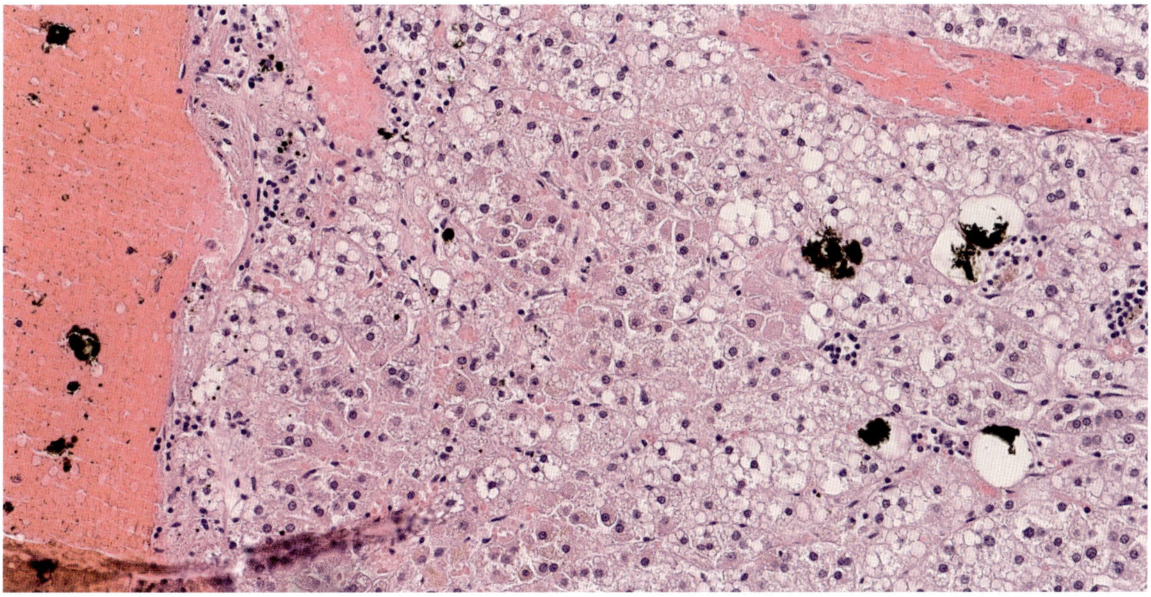

Fig. 7a3 Adrenal gland – Deposits: Case 17 (83y f, case report p. 82)
Crystalloide deposits of uncertain origin appearing black both in the parenchyma and in a vessel. HE 200x.

8. Kidney

a) Vascular changes

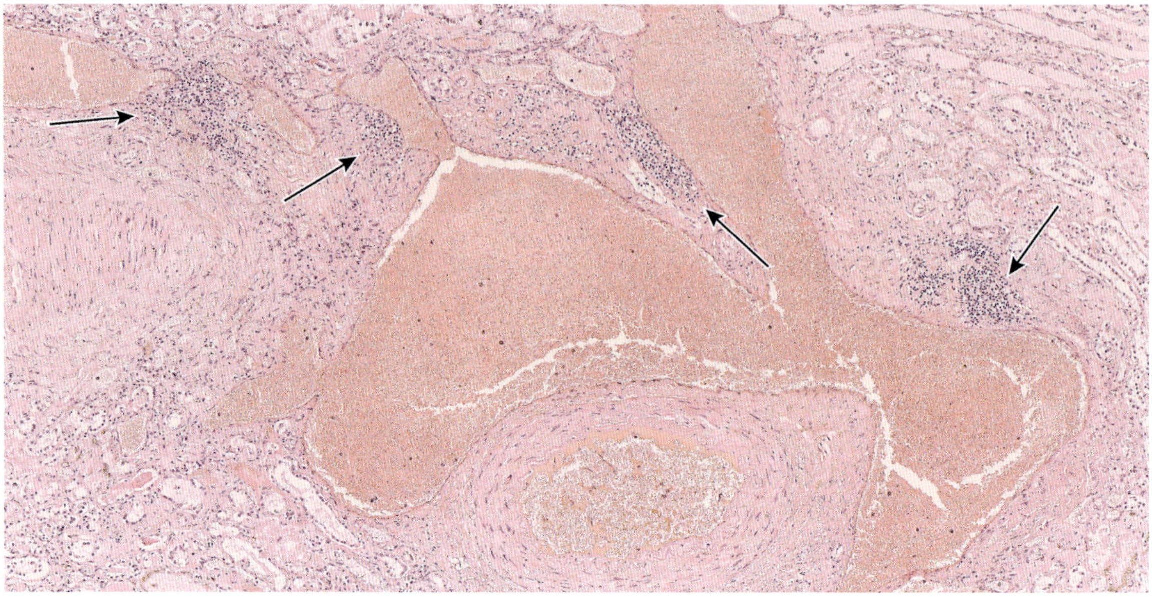

Fig. 8a1 Kidney – Vascular changes: Case 34 (79y m, case report p. 92)
Dense lymphocytic inflammatory infiltrates at several sites in the immediate vicinity of dilated venous vessels (arrows). HE 60x.

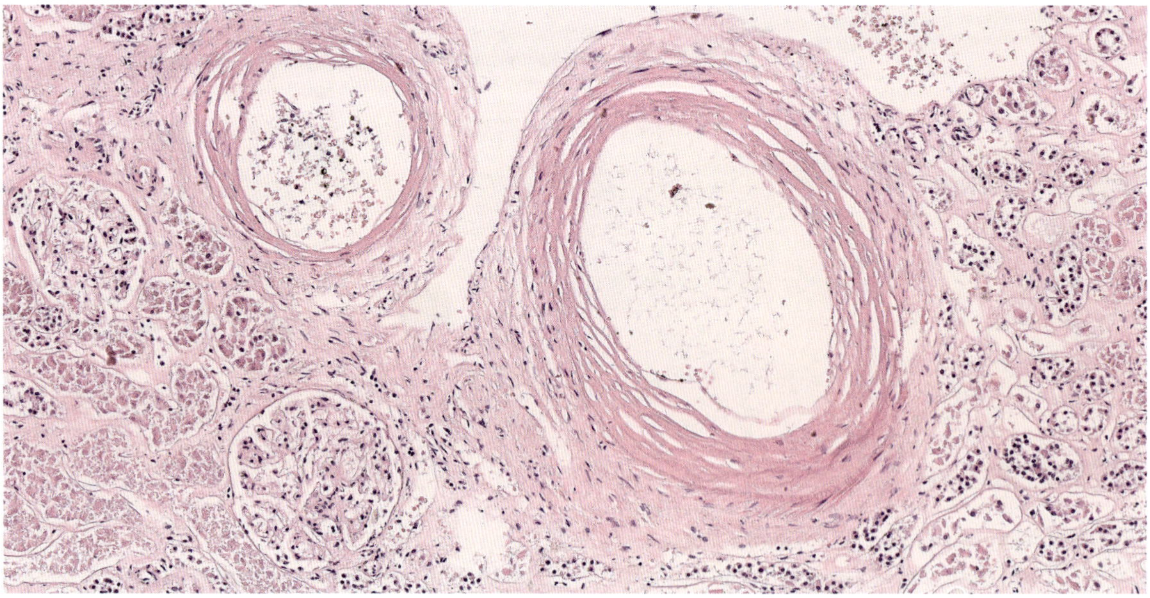

Fig. 8a2 Kidney – Vascular changes: Case 20 (59y f, case report p. 85)
Two smaller arterial vessels with oedematous loosened wall layers and the image of the so-called onion-skin pattern. HE 100x.

b) Deposits

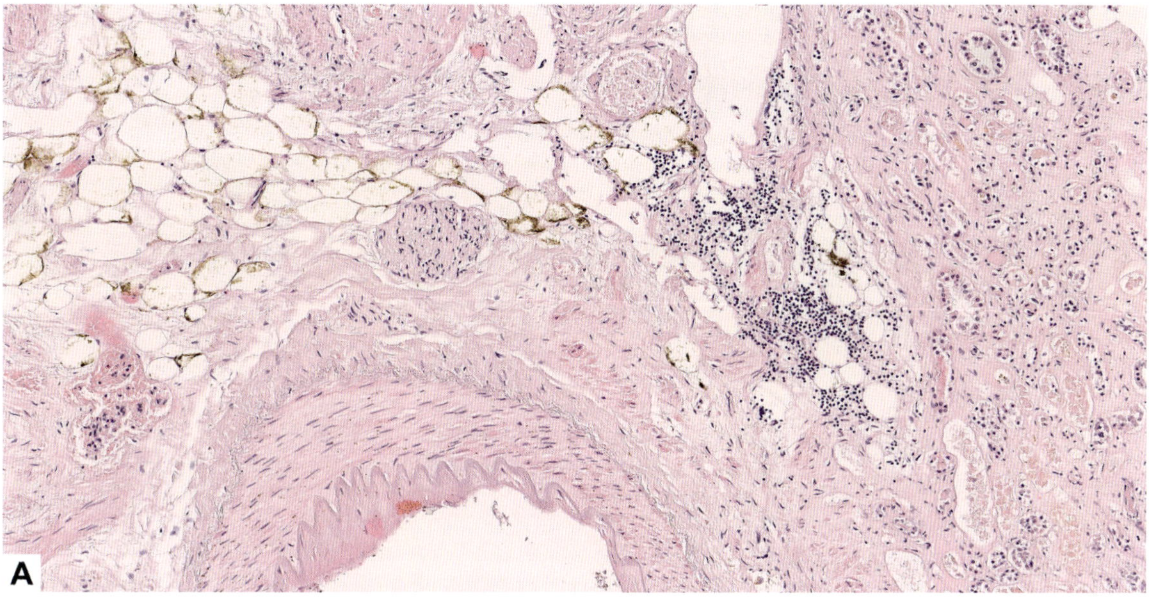

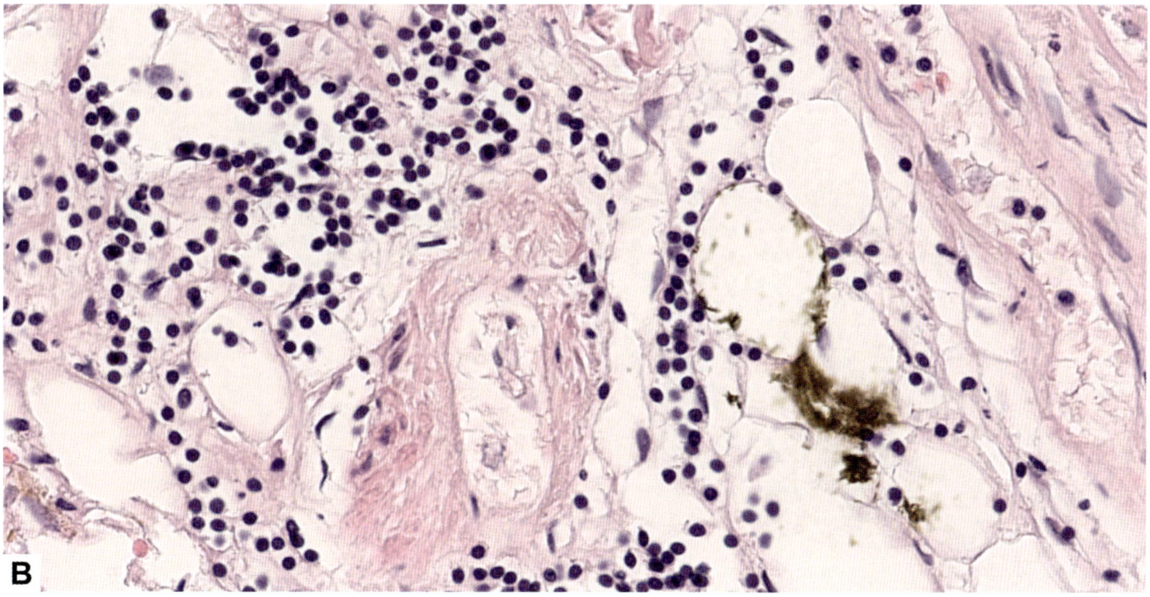

Fig. 8b Kidney – Deposits: Case 1 (82y f, case report p. 71)
A: Dark brown, crystalloide deposits of uncertain origin in numerous adipocytes in the fatty tissue of the renal pelvis. In addition, a patchy, inflammatory lymphocytic infiltrate. HE 100x.
B: Rod-shaped or needle-shaped brown-black appearing material. HE 500x.

9. Urinary bladder

a) Inflammatory changes

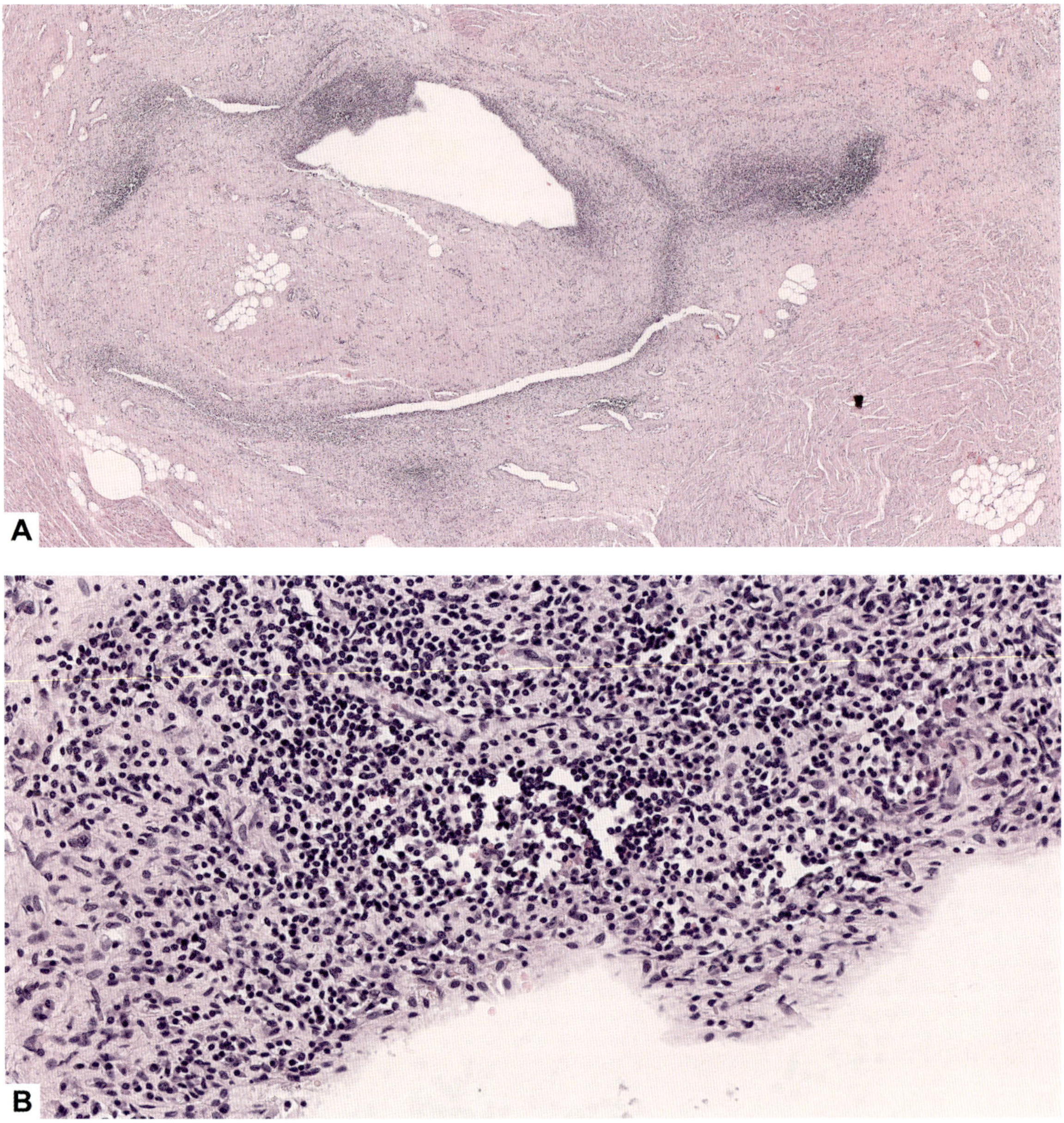

Fig. 9a Urinary bladder – Inflammatory changes: Case 19 (77y m, case report p. 84)
A: Ureteral ostium with distinct inflammatory infiltration. HE 100x.
B: Massive inflammatory lympho-plasmacellular infiltration in the area of the mucosa of the ureter. HE 200x.

10. Testis

a) Inflammatory changes

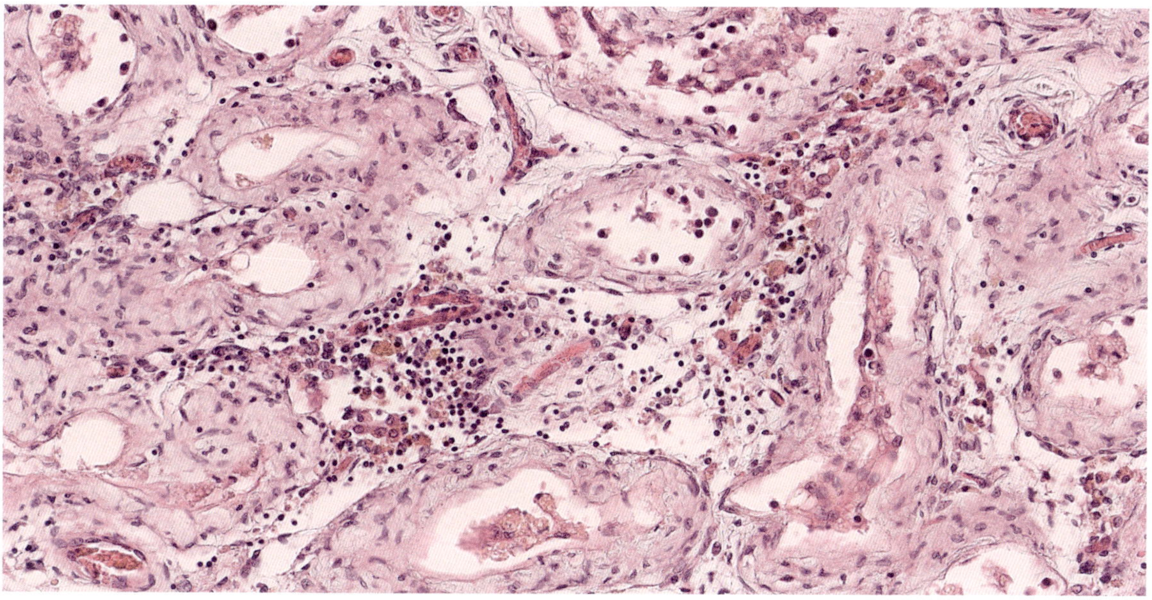

Fig. 10a Testis – Inflammatory changes: Case 56 (85y m, case report p. 98)
Perivascularly inflammatory cells consisting primarily of lymphocytes. HE 200x.

b) Spermatogenesis disorder

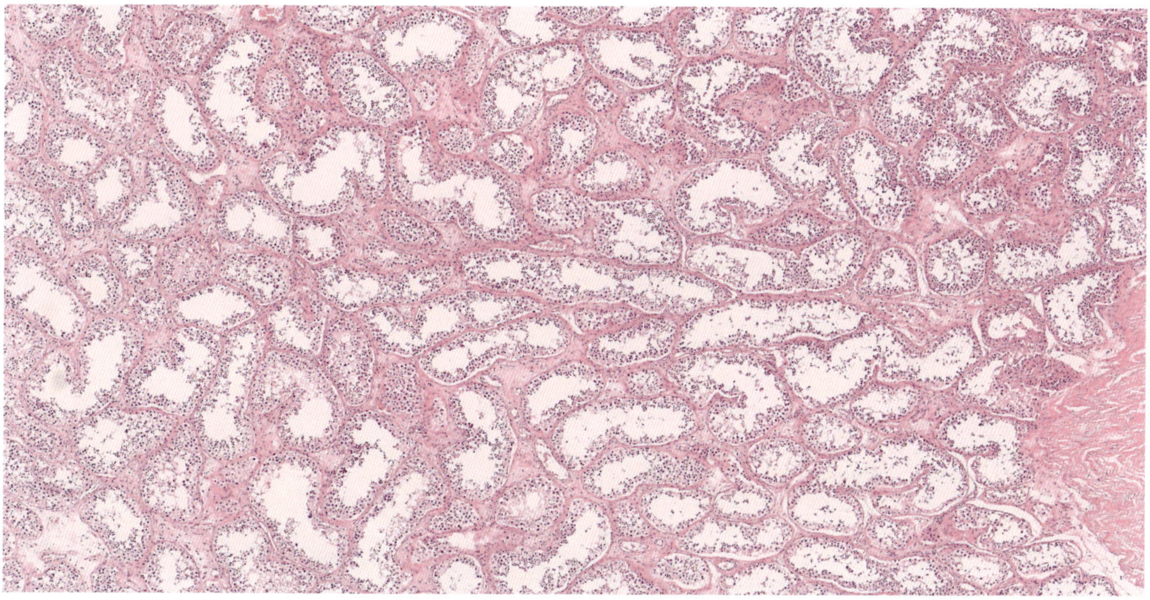

Fig. 10b Testis – Disorders of spermatogenesis: Case 18 (29y m, case report p. 83)
Significant reduction in spermatogenesis. HE 120x.

Continued on the next page.

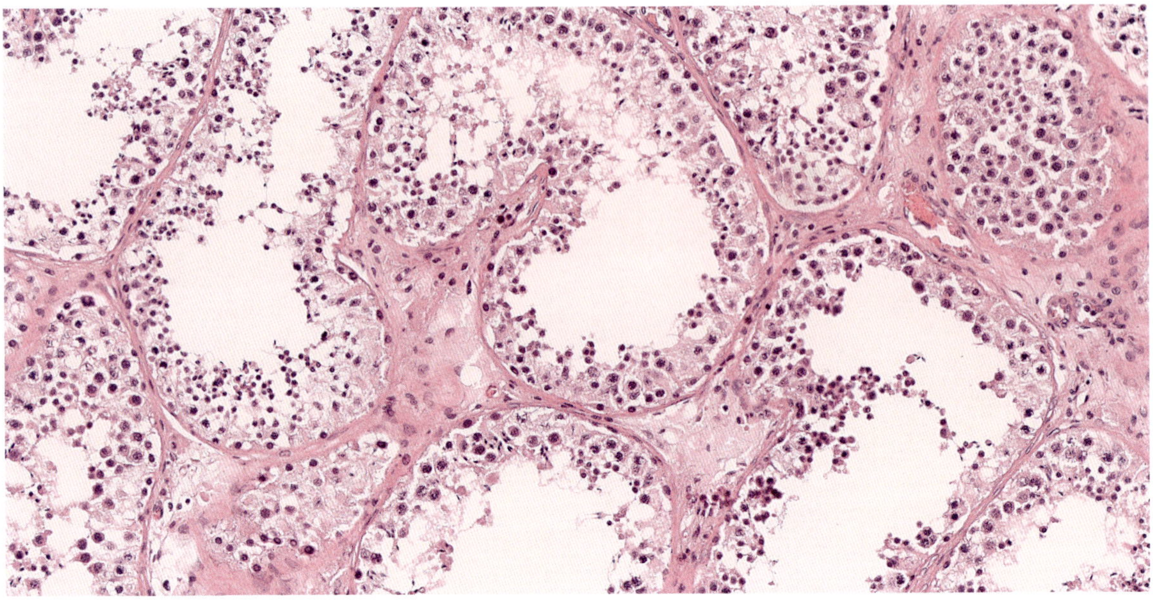

Fig. 10b Testis – Disorders of spermatogenesis: Continued case 18 (29y m, case report p. 83) Spermatogonia predominantly visible in the canaliculi and only very sparsely present spermatocytes and only very few spermatozoa. HE 160x.

11. Prostate

a) Inflammatory changes

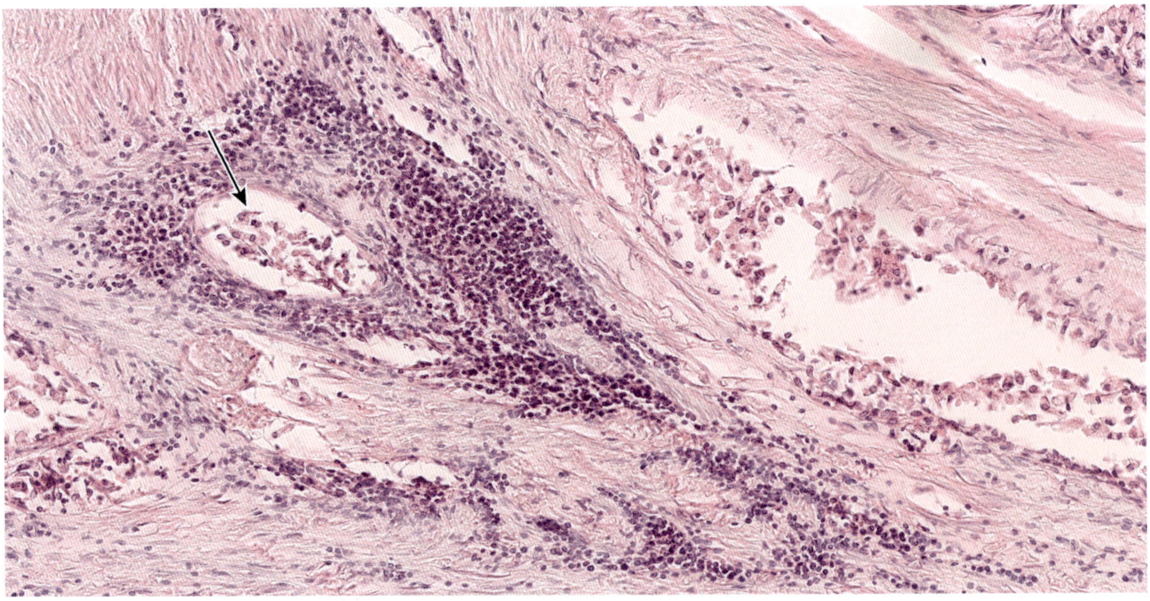

Fig. 11a Prostate – Inflammatory changes: Case 10 (61y m, case report p. 79) Massive perivascular infiltration and exfoliated endothelial cells in the vascular lumen (arrow) consistent with vasculitis. HE 190x.

12. Pancreas

a) Deposits

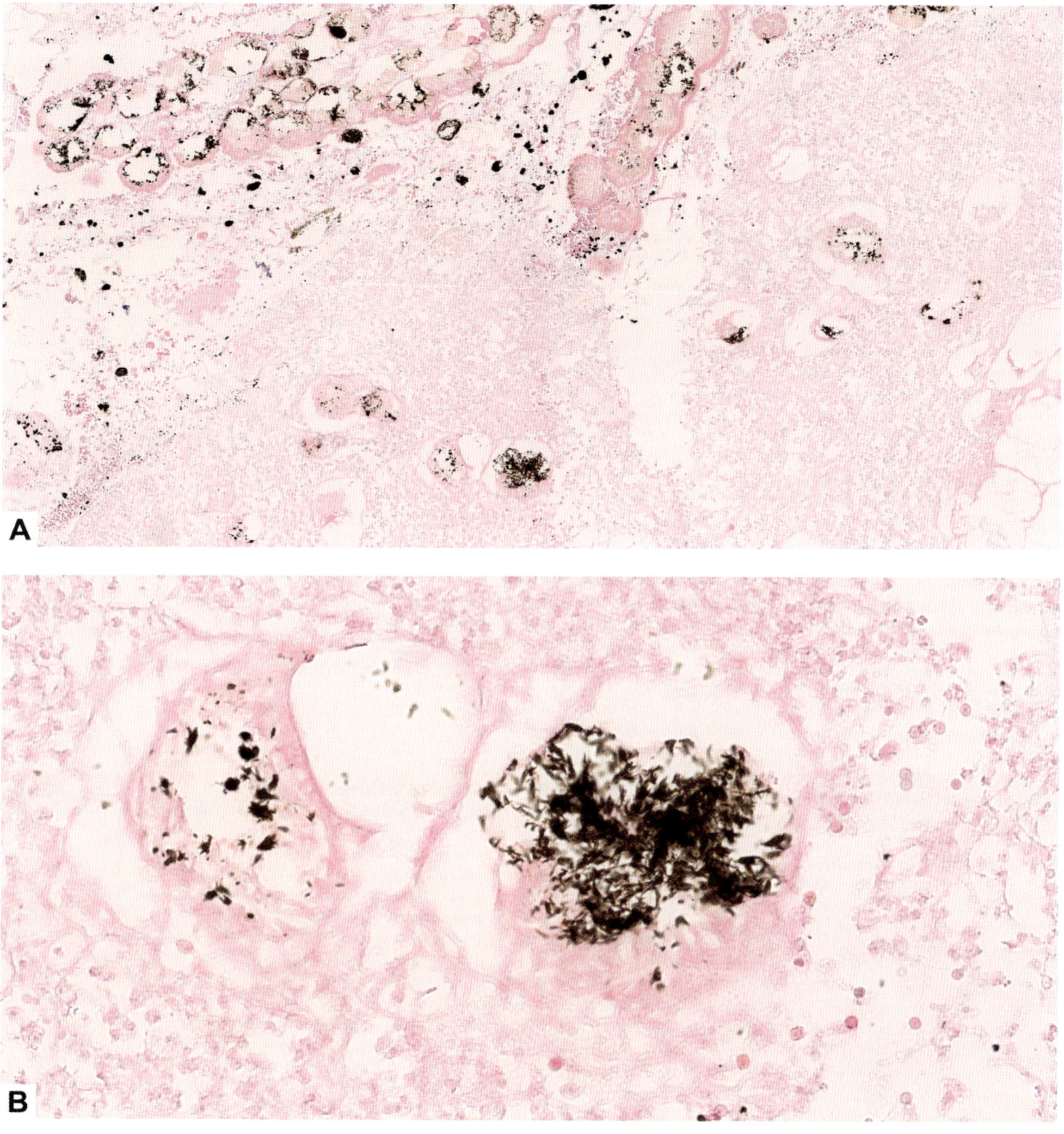

Fig. 12a Pancreas – Deposits: Case 13 (63y m, case report p. 81)
A: Both in the pancreatic parenchyma and in the peripancreatic fatty tissue in coarse vacuolar structures, abundant brown-black appearing crystalloide deposits of uncertain origin, fatty tissue necrosis and pronounced autolysis. HE 70x.
B: Coarse vacuolar structures with abundant brown-black, often rod-shaped, crystalloide material. HE 400x.

13. Peripheral nerves

a) Inflammatory changes

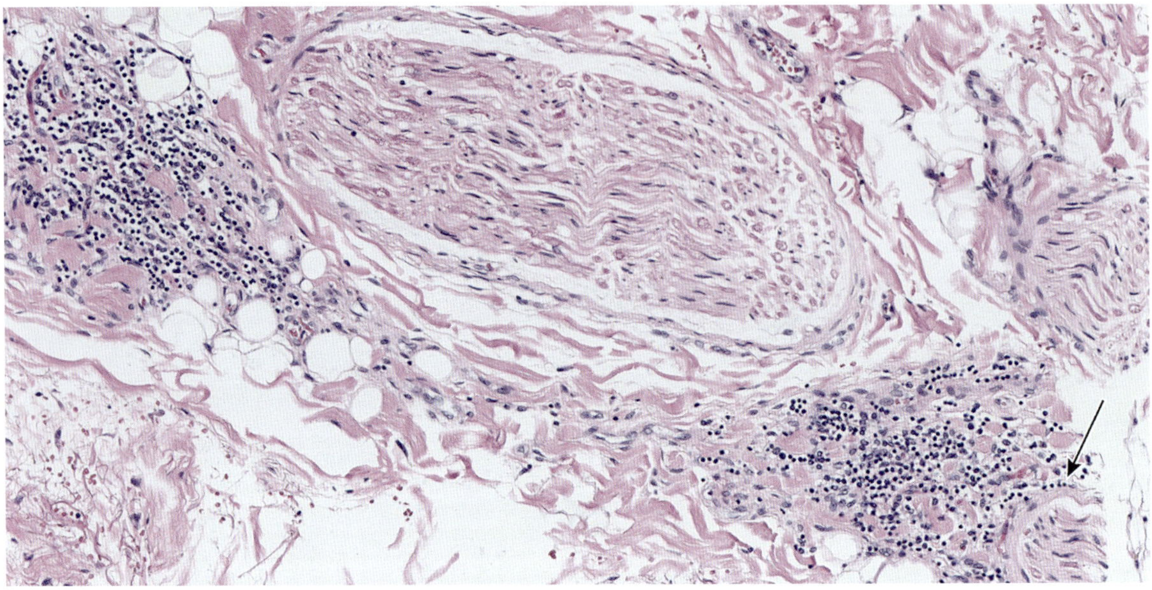

Fig. 13a Peripheral nerves – Inflammatory changes: External case (61y m, case report p. 125) Axillary nerve with patchy perineural lymphocytic infiltrate, partly in direct contact with the nerve (arrow). HE 140x.

14. Skeletal muscle

a) Inflammatory changes

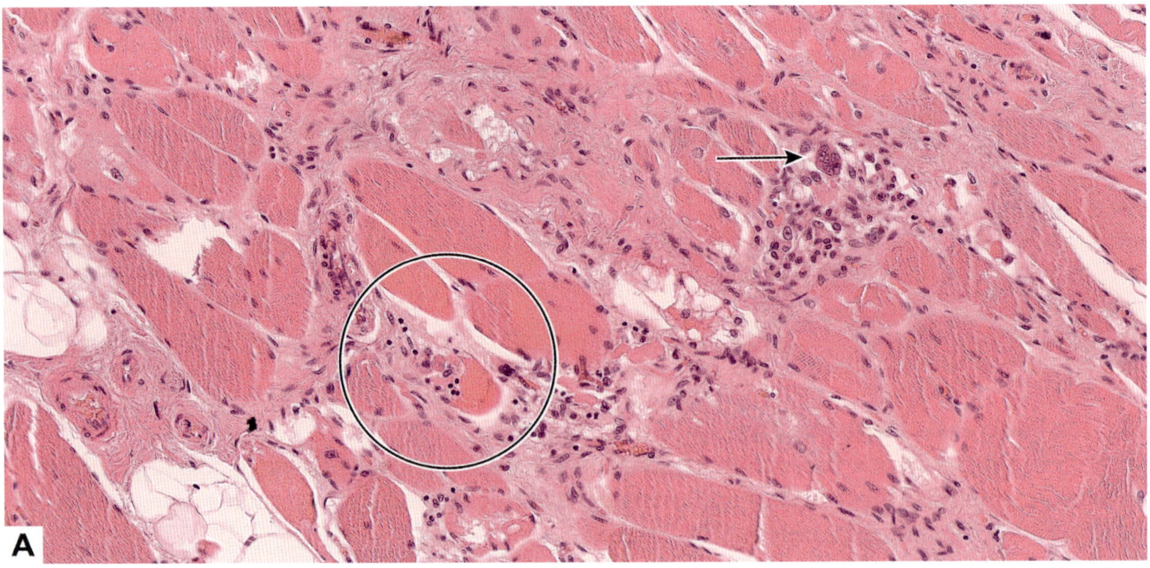

Fig. 14a Skeletal muscle – Inflammatory changes: Case 91 (74y m, case report p. 111)
A: Lower leg muscles with partial picture of acute myositis with lymphocyte infiltration and acute necrosis of a myocyte (circle), partial picture of an older inflammatory process with connective tissue-like transformation, histiocytic reaction including presence of a giant cell (arrow). HE 140x.

Continued on the next page.

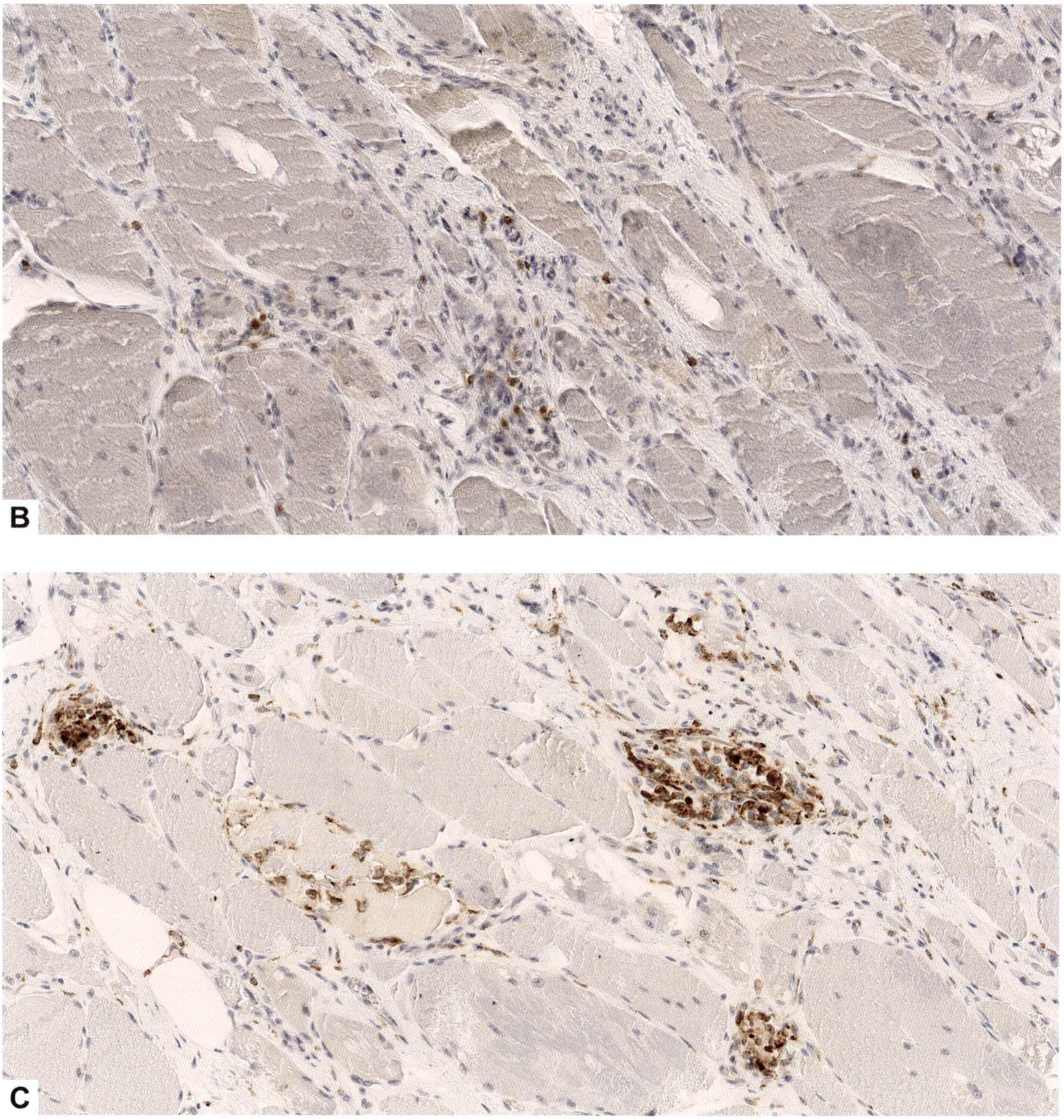

Fig. 14a Skeletal muscle – Inflammatory changes: Continued case 91 (74y m, case report p. 111)
B: In the immunohistochemical staining with CD3 patchy positivity, consistent with T lymphocytes. CD3 170x.
C: Clear positivity in immunohistochemical staining with CD68, consistent with a macrophagocytic infiltrate. CD68 170x.

b) Deposits

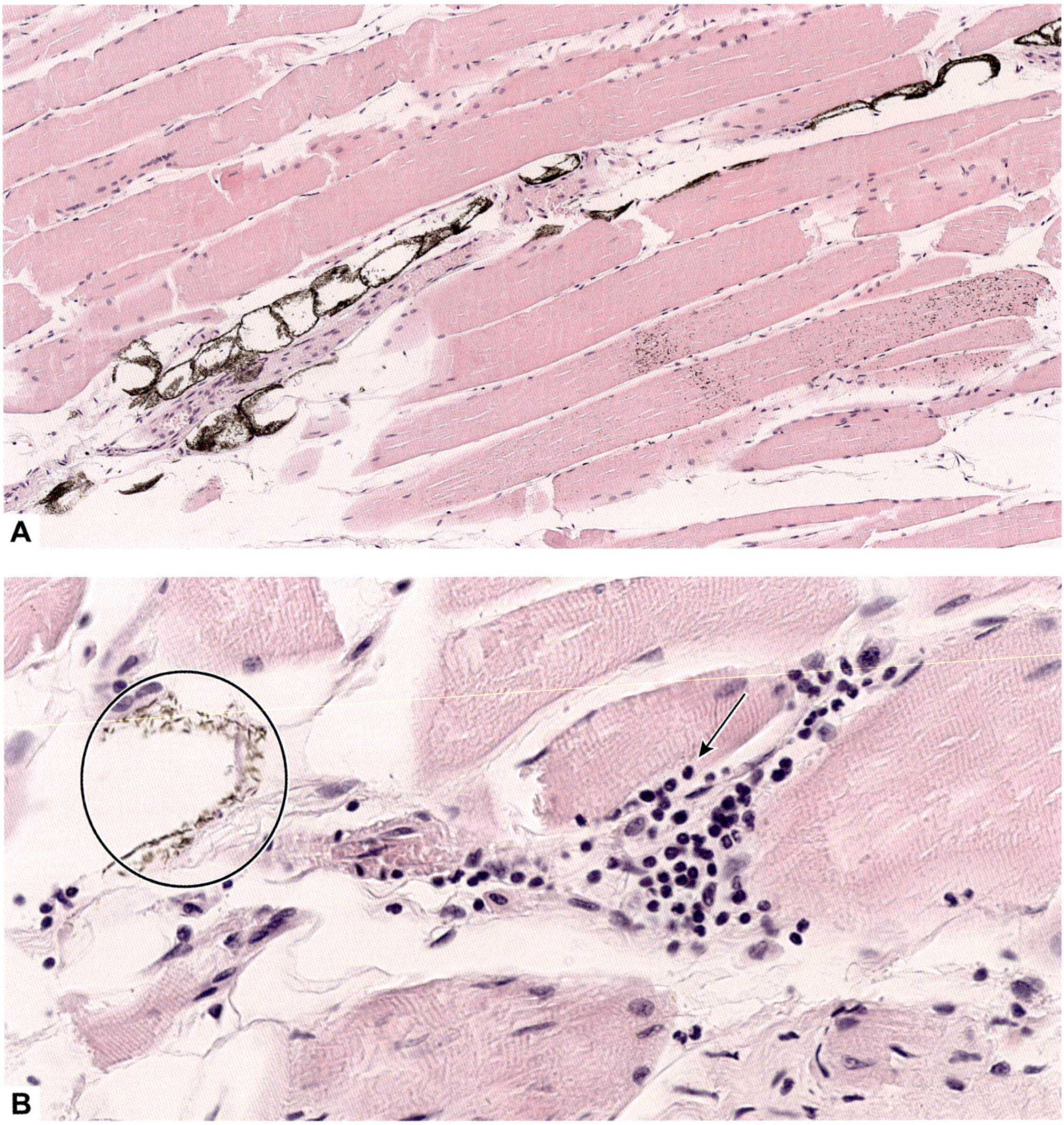

Fig. 14b Skeletal muscle – Deposits, inflammatory changes: Case 17 (83y f, case report p. 82)
A: Pronounced deposition of brown-black appearing crystalloide deposits of uncertain origin in the adipocytes. HE 110x.
B: Subtle deposition of dark brown, rod-shaped material in an adipocyte (circle), focal myositis with lymphocytic infiltrate, which partially spreads to the myocytes (arrow). HE 440x.

Case reports

1. Autopsies

82y / f / 2x Mod / 75, 40 **C1**

History of death and vaccination

The 82-year-old woman was found dead in the evening on 9 June 2021 by neighbours in her mid-terrace house in her bedroom bed, sitting sideways, slumped back on her back.

1st vaccination on 26 March 2021 with Moderna 3000495, death 75 days later
2nd vaccination on 30 April 2021 with Moderna 3000495, death 40 days later
On 24 April 2021 (29 days after the 1st vaccination) she had an unstoppable nose-bleed overnight and was taken to hospital by her son, where the bleeding was stopped by sclerotherapy.
On 22 May 2021 (24 days after the 2nd vaccination) she again had unstoppable nose bleeds overnight and was taken to hospital by her son, where this again was stopped by sclerotherapy.
On 9 June 2021 (40 days after the 2nd vaccination dose) she died at home. The son asked the doctor carrying out the post-mortem examination to arrange for a forensic medical examination.

Medical history

For about 2 months before her death, both legs of the 82-year-old woman had been very swollen following a wasp sting. She was a Marcumar patient due to atrial fibrillation. On 13 April 2021 she saw a gastroenterologist as she had previously lost weight. Due to impaired lung function, she was taking Salbutamol and using a breathing trainer.

Post-mortem examination (forensic medicine)

According to the forensic autopsy, the cause of death was suspected to be rhythmogenic heart failure and aspiration of food residues due to chronic cardiac stress caused by pulmonary sclerosis.

Post-mortem examination (pathology)

Cause of death: suspected heart failure due to chronic ischaemic myocardial disease
Main findings: Chronic obstructive pulmonary disease. Chronic bronchiolitis. Severe anthracosis. Fine-bubbling, partly also coarse-bubbling chronic-substantial pulmonary emphysema.

Secondary pathohistological examination

Lymphocytic infiltrates, partly nodular, were found in the lung, kidney and dura. There was no evidence of significant pre-existing myocardial lesions, but there was pronounced lymphocytic myocarditis and epicarditis.

In addition to the myocarditis, further COVID-19 vaccine-associated tissue changes were found: endothelialitis and focal obstructive vasculitis as well as lymphocytic alveolitis. Microemboli were found in the lungs, presumably with lipid-cholesterol materials, as indicated by inflammatory reactions with macrophages and foreign body giant cell formation around cholesterol formations.

Multiple non-localised, dark brown fibrous particle deposits were found in the lungs, heart and kidneys and in the periadrenal fatty tissue.

Such deposits are repeatedly seen in people who have died after COVID-19 vaccination. It has not yet been possible to clarify the composition and formation of these deposits. It is also not known whether they are of pathogenetic significance or may even have been involved in the death process. Immunohistochemical labelling of the S1 subunit of the spike protein (protein that the body's cells are forced to produce by COVID-19 vaccinations) was found in the myocytes of the heart muscle and in the endothelial cells of the vascular walls of all organs examined – from the aortic wall to the small vessels of the brain.

Spike protein expression in the ovaries is irrelevant for the death event, but is remarkable for gaining knowledge about the pathophysiological effects of the COVID-19 vaccinations, also with regard to a possible reduction in fertility. In this case, it is known that the deceased had given birth to two sons during her lifetime.

These COVID-19 vaccine-typical findings suggest several pathomechanisms leading to death:

Myocarditis can disrupt the conduction system of the heart and lead to cardiac arrest. This would fit in with the rhythmogenic heart failure diagnosed by the autopsy pathologist as the cause of death.

The **microemboli in the lungs** in the presence of foreign body particles, cholesterol formations and associated inflammation with foreign body giant cells may have led to an increase in pressure in the pulmonary circulation with subsequent **right heart failure.**

The episodes of unstoppable nose-bleeds in the Marcumar patient occurring 3 to 4 weeks after each of the COVID-19 vaccinations indicate a coagulation disorder. The COVID-19-vaccine-induced immune thrombotic thrombocytopenia (VITT) observed after COVID-19 vaccinations results in an increased tendency to bleed and an increased **tendency to thrombosis.**

It was probably a combination of myocarditis and an increased tendency to thrombosis with right side heart strain that ultimately led to heart failure.

A connection between the two COVID-19 vaccinations that took place and the death is **highly probable.**

71y / m / 1x Com / 31

History of death and vaccination

The 71-year-old man died on 1 May 2021, sitting in the driver's seat of his car to have a rest, after working with his wife in the forest.

1st vaccination on 31 March 2021 with Comirnaty ET3874, death 31 days later

He had been taking antihypertensives and lipid-lowering drugs (Ezetrol, Sortis) for years. He had an open leg wound above the right inner ankle for years and had worn anti-thrombosis stockings on both legs for decades.

Although the wife did not know about the vaccination plan on 31 March, she reported that she remembered the day because her husband came home unusually early. According to the vaccination sticker, the vaccination was administered on 31 March at 11:19 am. In the early evening on the day of the vaccination, he was sitting on the sofa in front of the television and suddenly spoke in a confused manner when talking to his wife. She then asked him specifically: "Is there something wrong with you?" He shook his head to indicate that there was nothing wrong with him. In the period that followed, he complained more and more often about his lack of appetite.

Post-mortem examination (forensic medicine)

During the autopsy, a pronounced hypertrophy of the heart was found (644 g, well above the so-called critical heart weight of 500 g, normal around 300 g). Bilateral endocardial fibrosis was found; no myocardial infarction scars. Moderate generalised arteriosclerosis. Pronounced acute congestive hyperaemia with oedema of the internal organs and brain.

The autopsy findings are seen as consistent with long-standing hypertension. The **cause of death** is considered to be rhythmogenic heart pump failure with significant cardiac antecedent disease (significant hypertrophy).

Secondary pathohistological examination

Features of typical coronavirus-induced organ and vascular lesions included focal **myocarditis, vascular inflammation with media necrosis** and predominantly **lymphocytic alveolitis/interstitial pneumonia.** In the brain there were features of recurrent micro haemorrhages due to small inflammatory vascular damage with massive haemosiderin deposits intra- and perivascularly. These explain the symptoms (confusion) on the evening of the vaccination, whereby the brain damage could initially be compensated for. On the day of death, **cerebral vascular lesions** were almost certainly the cause of death. However, the acute lesions could not be detected in the brain samples provided, especially as acute ischaemic brain tissue necrosis can only be reliably detected several hours after the event.

No spike protein could be detected immunohistochemically in the myocardium. In the prostate, however, there was a clear immunohistochemical display of (brown) spike protein. In the spleen, numerous scattered cell nuclei and the cytoplasm indicating anti-spike S1 antibodies.

In summary, the inflammatory vascular damage that typically occurs after COVID-19 vaccinations was found generalised in sections of various organs, including the brain. A (co-) causational reason of death by the COVID-19 vaccination is **probable.**

C3

94y / f / 1x Com, 1x UNKN / 125, 67

History of death and vaccination

The 94-year-old died on 9 June 2021 in her accommodation for assisted living.

1st vaccination on 4 February 2021 with Comirnaty, batch number unknown, death 125 days later

2nd vaccination on 3 April 2021 with UNKNOWN, death 67 days later

After the 1st dose, the general condition had deteriorated. Three days later there was a rapid deterioration with insufficient intake of food and fluids. In consultation with the daughter and in accordance with the patient's living will, palliative therapy was initiated. After the 2nd dose, there was initially no further deterioration.

Medical history

The 94-year-old woman had limited wheelchair mobility and lived in an assisted living facility. She had broken her femoral neck four years previously and had bruised her left arm once many years ago, which is why skin had been transplanted from her thigh to her arm.

Autopsy (forensic medicine)

Cause of death: Right-sided heart failure in the presence of a pulmonary infarction and clot occlusion of a pulmonary artery in a deep vein thrombosis. The onset of death may have been hurried up by the high-grade coronary artery calcification and the effusion in the thoracic cavities.

"From a forensic medical point of view, there is no connection with the vaccination that was given more than two months ago."

Secondary pathohistological examination

Vascular alterations were found, which are repeatedly observed in people who have died after coronavirus vaccinations: Media necrosis, perivasculitis also in pulmonary arteries.

A **pulmonary infarction** found was not quite recent and may have contributed significantly to the death due to **the right heart problems,** but did not directly cause it.

In several organs there was a picture of obliterating **vasculitis of small vessels with lymphocytic inflammation** and **amyloid-like deposits.** Minimal **myocarditis.**

In the heart, lungs, kidneys and pancreas we found **darkly pigmented, granular particle deposits,** which is often found in people who have died after COVID-19 vaccination. The origin, development and pathogenetic significance of these deposits is still unclear.

The expression of the spike protein, which the COVID-19 vaccinations induce the body cells to produce, was detected immunohistochemically in the aortic wall, between the elastic lamellae, nuclear, perinuclear and also in the area of cystic lesions.

Judgement in this case is made with the restriction that the brain was not examined.

The vascular changes and also focal deposits of non-localised material speak in favour of a significant role of the COVID-19 vaccinations in the multifactorial death process.

A connection between the death and the COVID-19 vaccination is therefore **probable.**

C4

75y / f / 1x Com / xx

History of death and vaccination

The 75-year-old woman died on 1 June 2021 in the intensive care unit after hospitalisation due to "unclear somnolence". Sepsis with an unclear focus was treated.
A reminder card from Biontech/Pfizer for the "2nd vaccination" on 16 June 2021 was found in her home, from which it was concluded that a first vaccination must have been given. According to the family, the vaccination card was "no longer up to date". The family doctor's practice refused to provide information about the first vaccination, citing data protection.
1st vaccination with Comirnaty, date and batch number unknown
Pre-existing disease was a minimal arteriosclerosis and, according to clinical information, a high-grade mitral and tricuspid valve insufficiency.

Autopsy (forensic medicine)

Cause of death was sepsis with an unclear starting point of infection.

Secondary pathohistological examination

There was no evidence of sepsis, in particular no abscessing pyelonephritis. However, there was evidence of vaccine-induced damage in several organs: mild **myocarditis** with inflammation of the vessels in the myocardium was found in the heart muscle. In the arteries of the spleen, **elastic destruction** with focal gap formation in the larger splenic arteries was found. The splenic arterioles and arteries showed a clear onion skin phenomenon – a typical vascular damage pattern after COVID-19 vaccinations. In the liver and especially in the spleen, signs of mesenteric artery or portal vein thrombosis were found. In the liver, canalicular bilirubin thrombus deposits were found centrally in zone 1 of the lobes. The spleen was necrotic, but not autolytic, but intravitally necrotised, probably as a result of the aforementioned mesenteric artery or portal vein thrombosis, to which the liver findings with the bilirubin deposits also correspond.
The expression of the spike protein, which the COVID-19 vaccinations cause the body cells to produce, was detected in the skin. Here, a Spike-S1-labeled antibody revealed proven immunohistochemical nuclear and perinuclear markings in basal and suprabasal cells as well as in the endothelia of small vessels.
Suspicious looking, amyloid-like deposits are found in the walls of small vessels intracerebrally, in the skin and perivascularly in the lungs.
Necrosis of the spleen, pancreas and liver, as we found in **mesenteric or portal vein thrombosis,** is in the foreground. The associated shock was probably the cause of death. The thrombosis was probably caused by vasculitis, which was detected in the organs described above.
A connection between vaccination and death seems **very likely** in view of the pronounced vascular damage typical of COVID-19 vaccination.

C7

57y / m / 2x Com / 48, 7

History of death and vaccination

The 57-year-old died on 1 May 2021.

1st vaccination on 25 March 2021 with Comirnaty EY7015, death 48 days later
2nd vaccination on 5 May 2021 with Comirnaty FD4555, death 7 days later
An autopsy was carried out in the pathology department of the hospital. As this was a forensic medical autopsy, only sparse information was made available to the autopsy examiner.

Post-mortem examination (forensic medicine)

The autopsy revealed a male corpse in normal nutritional condition. The skin of the thorax showed some stroma marks (after resuscitation). The lymph nodes at the bronchial bifurcation were anthracotic. The heart was slightly larger than the corpse's fist, 480 g. Intima plaques in coronary arteries with stenosis of up to 60 %. Posterior wall infarction with a 10 x 10 mm yellow-pale area.
Cause of death: Acute myocardial infarction in the posterior wall of the left ventricle.
Underlying disease: Coronary sclerosis.
Individual anatomical diagnoses:

- Stenosing coronary sclerosis
- Acute myocardial infarction in the posterior wall of the left ventricle
- Acute pulmonary congestion
- Liver congestion 1st degree

Secondary pathohistological examination

The typical picture of an ischaemic myocardial infarction due to coronary sclerosis or thrombosis was not present.
Mild lymphocytic epicarditis and foci of **lymphocytic myocarditis** with necrosis were found in the heart.
The typical features of **vascular inflammation of the aorta with media necrosis** and dissection were present, which is repeatedly observed in people who have died after COVID-19 vaccination.
The secondary examination was limited due to the fact that only the microscopic section preparations were available, but no tissue samples were available. Further investigations using special staining or immunohistochemical methods were therefore not possible.
A connection between the two performed COVID-19 vaccinations and the death is **highly probable.**

C8

78y / m / 1x Com / 35

Death and vaccination history

The 78-year-old male died on 18 July 2021.

1st vaccination on 6 May 2021 with Comirnaty, batch number unknown, death 35 days later

Post-mortem examination (forensic medicine)

The body of a 78-year-old man weighing 97.5 kg and 176 cm tall was found.

Cause of death: Acute anterior wall infarction of the heart showing recurrent myocardial infarctions, very severe heart enlargement and myocardial scarring (callous heart) due to myocardial infarction.

Generalised calcification of the arteries, numerous calcification zones and ruptured vessel walls of the large body arteries.

Advanced calcification with constricting calcification of the coronary arteries. Stenosis in the anterior branch by 75 %. No fresh or old clot deposits. Heart weight 725 g, left wall thickness approx. 2 cm. Signs of atrial fibrillation: Dilatation and endocardial fibrosis in the left atrium.

Repeated myocardial infarctions: Extensive infarction scar in the area of the left posterior wall of the heart (6 x 4 cm). Minor scarring close to the base in the anterior wall of the left ventricle. Patchy and striated scarring of the anterior and posterior cylindrical inner heart muscle – Several days to weeks old infarct areas with gelatinous, reddish granulation tissue showing in the anterior wall of the left ventricle (2 x 1 cm) as well as adjacent to the posterior wall infarct (2 x 2 cm) – Acute, slightly clay-coloured, blistered anterior heart wall infarct (5 x 3 cm; extending to the left-side ventricular edge area).

Signs of acute bi-ventricular heart failure, leading to left ventricular failure: dilatation of the cardiac cavities. Liquid blood in the corpse. Generalised cyanosis. Congestive haemorrhage and hyperaemia of the lung tissue. Chronic obstructive pulmonary disease (COPD). Heavy carbon deposits in the lung tissue (anthracosis).

Secondary pathohistological examination

There are clear signs of vascular damage **(endothelialitis)** in several organs; in some cases deposits of amyloid-like material, textural disorders of the pulmonary artery with lymphocytic infiltrates. Multiple non-localised vacuolar deposits, in many areas, but mainly in the lungs. Such deposits and vascular damage are typically found following a COVID-19 vaccination.

Coronary artery sclerosis is only moderate. In the myocardium only moderate scarring and no clear signs of recent myocardial infarction. **Lymphocytic myocarditis** in conjunction with intracardiac vaccine-induced vascular damage must be considered as a contributing factor to death.

However, spike protein expression could not be detected in the organ tissues examined (lung, spleen, liver), so that involvement of the COVID-19 vaccination consequences must only be regarded as probable. The pathohistological appearance of inflamed vessel walls is quite typical, as is repeatedly seen after COVID-19 vaccinations.

Since our second examination was only microscopic, we were of course unable to assess the anterior wall infarction visible in the first autopsy, although the pathohistological picture did not impress us as a classic infarction scenario. However, infarct genesis with thrombus formation on inflamed inner coronary vessel walls is conceivable. A connection between vaccination and death seems **likely** due to the myocarditis and COVID-19 vaccine-typical vascular damage.

C9

89y / f / 1x UNKN / approx. 182

History of death and vaccination

The 89-year-old woman died on 11 August 2021, about 6 months after the coronavirus vaccination. Unfortunately, no vaccination documentation was available.

1st vaccination: early 2021 with UNKNOWN vaccine status, death approx. 182 days later

The 89-year-old woman was admitted to the hospital as an emergency in a state of shock with multiple organ failures. She had eaten and drunk little in the period prior to the event; weight loss of approx. 20 kg within 3 to 4 months. X-ray of the abdomen shows a mirror image.

Autopsy (pathology) – cause of death: fresh thrombosis of the superior mesenteric artery, which led to mesenteric ischaemia. The patient died in shock with multiple organ failure. Pre-existing severe generalised arteriosclerosis.

Secondary pathohistological examination

The shock event leading to death was triggered by a thrombotic **occlusion of the superior mesenteric artery,** which led to subtotal intestinal necrosis. This mesenteric thrombosis is probably not solely due to the atherosclerosis of these arteries, but is probably also caused by the media necrosis and dissection of the mesenteric arteries.

This vascular damage is not isolated. Rather, **vascular wall damage with deposits of hyaline amyloid like material** is also found in the vessels of the heart and lungs. Such vascular damage, especially mesenteric vascular thrombosis, fits the now familiar picture of inflammatory vascular damage found in people who have died after COVID-19 vaccinations. It therefore seems very likely that these COVID-19 vaccination-related vascular inflammations were involved in the death.

As there were no paraffin-embedded tissue samples available, it was not possible to carry out any examinations beyond the light microscopic examination of the available sectional preparations, such as special staining or immunohistochemical examinations, especially with regard to the spike protein S1. This evidence could provide further proof of a connection between COVID-19 vaccination, thrombi and death. Histological sections of the brain were not available.

A connection between the death and the COVID-19 vaccination that took place, is **very likely.**

C10

61y / m / 2x Com / 67, 25

History of death and vaccination

The 61-year-old died in his home on 31 August 2021.

1st vaccination on 25 June 2021 with Comirnaty 1D017A, death 67 days later
2nd vaccination on 6 August 2021 with Comirnaty FF3318, death 25 days later

The 61-year-old man complained of sudden chest pain and collapsed on 31 August 2021 while having breakfast with his partner. He was resuscitated by his partner and then by the emergency team, but no spontaneous circulation could be established. On admission to the emergency department, echocardiography revealed an already coagulated pericardial tamponade.

Medical history

- Myocarditis 30 years ago following a flu-like infection
- High blood pressure medication
- Lots of coffee, smoked a lot
- Retired 2 years ago, previously self-employed
- 1.76 m, 90 kg
- COVID-19 vaccinations because he wanted to travel to Turkey
- 3 weeks after the 1st vaccination, "fell off his chair" while on holiday at the North Sea with his partner, ambulance, hospital. Nothing was found and "dehydration" was given as the reason for the collapse
- Bladder infection shortly before death

Autopsy (pathology)

Cause of death: pericardial tamponade due to aortic rupture at the bottom of an aortic aneurysm. There was a high-grade general arteriosclerosis, a dissection of the ascending aorta and the aortic arch with consecutive wall rupture of the ascending aorta at the pericardial envelope of 3.2 cm length and 0.4 cm diameter as well as a haemorrhagic pericardial tamponade. In addition, there was a high-grade coronary arteriosclerosis and a high-grade cardiac hypertrophy and dilatation.

Secondary pathohistological examination

In the total of 26 organ samples, typical COVID-19 vaccination-associated organ changes were found in addition to age-appropriate changes: minor endothelialitis in the heart muscle, minor pericarditis, focal myocarditis.

In addition to the undoubtedly present atherosclerotic changes, the available sectional preparations show a profound **textural disorder of the aorta with media necrosis,** dissection, destruction of elastic layers, focal dense inflammatory infiltrations and considerable perivascular inflammation of the vasa vasorum.

Lymphocytic infiltrates outside the lymphatic organs, particularly in the testicles and epididymis, lungs, kidneys and spleen. In the spleen, the typical onion skin-like loosening of the vessel walls with clear expression of spike protein is particularly impressive. Also diffuse throughout the spleen parenchyma.

Hepatocytes do not express spike protein, but vascular wall cells of intrahepatic vessels do. The overall histological findings in conjunction with the spike protein immunohistochemistry prove that the patient had pronounced coronavirus vaccine-induced organ changes, in particular an excessive immune reaction. The cause of death, as already established in the initial autopsy, was clearly a **dissection of the ascending aorta with wall rupture** and haemorrhage. The deep-seated media necrosis of the aortic wall points towards a possible inflammatory toxic genesis. In fact, the spike protein was detected in the aortic wall in myofibroblasts in inflammatory cells and also perivascularly around the vasa vasorum.
The histological picture does not correspond to the usual atherosclerotic dissection with rupture. An idiopathic microcystic medianecrosis or a chronic inflammatory disease can be excluded with certainty.
It is **almost certain** that there is a connection between the COVID-19 vaccinations that took place and the death.

C12

81y / f / 1x Com / 23
History of death and vaccination
The 81-year-old died on 22 May 2021 at 10:13 pm in the presence of her brother.
1st vaccination on 29 April 2021 with Comirnaty EX3599, death 23 days later
The 81-year-old had called her brother because of severe chest pains. On the way to his car to go to hospital, she collapsed. She had previously refused resuscitation.
According to her daughter and granddaughter, who suspected that the death was a result of the coronavirus vaccination, the deceased was "in top form". They filed a complaint against the family doctor who vaccinated her. The doctor pointed out previous illnesses, but was also surprised by the death, as the woman still was showing great vitality.

Medical history
According to the general practitioner, she suffered from the following pre-existing conditions: Hypertensive heart disease, high blood pressure, valvular heart disease, polyarthrosis, aortic ectasia and a right-sided shoulder end prosthesis. According to a doctor's letter dated 20 May 2019, she also had an ACE inhibitor-induced cough.

Post-mortem examination (forensic medicine)
There is a report from a chief police inspector who attended the post-mortem examination. According to this report, the post-mortem examiners found signs of chronic lung disease (COPD.) Her heart had a critical weight of (480 g). There was also insufficiency of the tricuspid valve and calcification of the coronary arteries. The cause of death was cardiac decompensation.
An autopsy report (abridged version) dated 4 June 2021 is also available. Here, moderate calcification of the aortic valve, moderate calcification of the coronary arteries, moderate calcification of the aorta and the blood vessels at the base of the

brain as well as hyperinflation of the lungs consistent with COPD and pulmonary hypertension are stated.
Cause of death: cardiac decompensation.

Secondary pathohistological examination
The textural disorders of the vascular wall layers found in the myocardium, spleen, kidney and cerebellum are repeatedly seen in people who have died after COVID-19 vaccinations.
Brownish fibrous particles were conspicuous in the myocardium, pancreas and cerebellum. Such deposits are repeatedly found in people who have died after coronavirus vaccination. It has not yet been possible to clarify the composition and origin of these deposits. It is also unknown whether they are of pathogenetic significance or may even have been involved in the death process.
Immunohistochemical positivity of the S1 subunit of the spike protein (protein that the body cells are forced to produce due to COVID-19 vaccinations) was found in the walls of intramural vessels of the heart muscle in endothelia and subendothelial in the area of hyaline swelling.
COVID-19 vaccine-typical damage was therefore found, which makes a causal relationship between the COVID-19 vaccination that took place and the death 23 days later **probable.**

63y / m / 1x Astra / 6 **C13**
History of death and vaccination
The 63-year-old died on 25 May 2021 at 7:15 am at work, where he received approx. 10 minutes of layman resuscitation, continued by an emergency physician for approx. 90 minutes under thrombolytic therapy. According to his wife, he went to work without symptoms.
1st **vaccination** on 19 May 2021 with Astra Zeneca ABX5182, death 6 days later

Medical history
According to the daughter, she had not noticed any symptoms of her father's heart disease and was somewhat surprised by the results of the autopsy. He was in good health for his age and had played sport. The family doctor reported a pre-existing high blood pressure, gout, elevated blood lipid levels, calcification of the aortic valve and increased curvature of the thoracic spine.

Autopsy (forensic medicine)
Cause of death:
- Acute left heart failure
- Reduced blood flow to the heart muscles due to coronary artery calcification
- Hypertensive heart disease

Myocardial infarction in the anterior descending branch with blood clot already in the process of breaking down. Acute left heart failure with pronounced congestion with pronounced coronary artery calcification and hypertensive heart disease, heart weight 517 g (critical upper limit heart weight from 500 g), pericardium firmly fused to the heart.

Secondary pathohistological examination
Pre-existing pronounced general athero- and coronary sclerosis. Myocardial callosities. According to forensic findings, extensive acute myocardial infarctions.
Dissection of the aorta and wall damage of larger vessels **with inflammatory reactions** are in the foreground. No perforations.
Remarkable is the massive scattering of **brownish fibrous particles** in almost all body organs, but not in the two examined sections of the brain. In the lungs, features of lipid pneumonia with foreign body giant cells and lymphocytic infiltrates consistent with endogenous allergic pneumonitis. The spike protein produced by the body cells as a result of the COVID-19 vaccinations could not be detected immunohistochemically.
Clear vaccine-associated organ damage was found, which certainly contributed significantly to the death from a recent heart attack.
The connection between the death and the vaccination seems **very likely** despite the fact that spike protein expression was not detectable.

C17

83y / f / 1x Com / 10
History of death and vaccination
The 83-year-old woman died on 16 April 2021 and was found dead in her bedroom by her neighbour.
1st vaccination on 6 April 2021 with Comirnaty, batch number unknown, death 10 days later

Medical history
Known high blood pressure, had not seen the family doctor for 5 years.
All findings unremarkable, "fit and mentally up to scratch". According to the neighbour, leg vein thrombosis.

Autopsy (forensic medicine)
Softening of the brain consistent with a stroke, which could be the cause of death. Acute softening of the left frontal brain measuring 4 x 3 x 2 cm. Black-red haemorrhage in the scalp of the right forehead. Severe sclerosis of the basal cerebral arteries and the large body arteries. Smallest calf vein thrombosis on the left. Slit-shaped foramen ovale.

Secondary pathohistological examination

COVID-19 vaccine-typical vascular damage was found in various organs, including in the coronary vessels in the form of media necrosis and in the spleen in the form of pronounced 'onion-skin-like' textural disorders of the splenic artery walls.

Perivascular lymphocytic inflammation was found in brain tissue, sometimes with endothelial swelling.

After vaccination, **black-brown, granular,** as yet unidentified **materials** were repeatedly found in the spleen, adrenal gland, heart, liver and skeletal muscle, but not in the lungs. So far, it has not been possible to clarify the origin, nature and potential significance of these materials for the occurrence of illness and death in people who died after COVID-19 vaccinations.

A connection between the death and the COVID-19 vaccination seems to exist with a **probability bordering on certainty.** This is supported by the immunohistochemical spike protein detection in myocardium and vascular endothelia.

29y / m / 1x Com, 1x Astra / 134, 46 **C18**

History of death and vaccination

Death on 6 July 2021 at the age of 29 years after seizure on the evening of 5 July 2021 and emergency admission to hospital.

1st vaccination on 22 February 2021 with Astra Zeneca ABV3025, death 134 days later
2nd vaccination on 21 May 2021 with Comirnaty EX3510, death 46 days later

On 5 July, the 29-year-old had a barbecue with his family during the day. According to reports from his relatives, he was in good health and had to lay down briefly afterwards due to a slight headache. Recently, he had often reported such mild headaches. The family (the deceased's young son and his partner) had sat together in the evening. As the deceased was on duty at the hospital quite early the next day, he had not drunk much. He had not taken any drugs. Late in the evening, he was found convulsing by his partner. Emergency doctor intervened with circulatory stabilisation.

The first hospital refused to admit him as the intensive care unit was full to capacity with coronavirus cases. He was then transferred to another hospital for internal intensive care. A broad drug and alcohol screening was negative, a bihemispheric subarachnoid haemorrhage was detected in the cranial CT scan. The patient was transferred to neurosurgery that same night. Brain death was diagnosed there.

Autopsy (pathology)

Cause of death: Central death due to subarachnoid haemorrhage. Heart largely normal, few signs of chronic, uncharacteristic myocarditis (CD15, CD3, CD20, CD68, CD4, CD8).

Secondary pathohistological examination

Subarachnoid haemorrhage is an obvious immediate **cause of death,** but it is difficult to determine its cause. A pathohistological examination by a specialist in neuro-

pathology, who looks impartially for possible damage caused by the COVID-19 vaccination in the brain, would be desirable.
There were signs of thrombus formation in various places in the brain tissue as well as traces of the subarachnoid haemorrhage that had taken place. **Perivascular lymphocytic inflammation** in the area of the **cerebral vessels,** partly with endothelial swelling. Vascular damage was found in various organs. Signs of mild focal **myocarditis** and pronounced lymphocytic endothelial inflammation of the myocardial vessels were found in the heart muscle, in some cases with destruction of the vessel wall.
Spike protein in the myocardial tissue, immunohistochemically isolated, perinuclear, slightly granular positive in about one third of the nuclei of myocytes, but also of interstitial cells.
Macrophage-rich **alveolitis** in the lungs and perivascular lymphocytic inflammation. Lymphocytic vascular inflammation was also found in the liver and spleen, particularly of the inner walls of the vessels, with onion-skin-like textural disorders of the vessel walls in the spleen. A secondary finding, irrelevant to the cause of death, was the pronounced expression of spike protein S1 in the area of the seminiferous tubules with a clear stratification disorder of spermatogenesis.
Due to the overall findings, in particular the strong expression of spike protein in some cases, there is a connection between COVID-19 vaccination and death with a **probability bordering on certainty.**

C19

77y / m / 2x Com / 124, 82

History of death and vaccination

The 77-year-old died on 17 August 2021 after a two-week stay in hospital.
1st vaccination on 15 April 2021 with Comirnaty, batch number unknown, death 124 days later
2nd vaccination on 27 May 2021 with Comirnaty, batch number unknown, death 82 days later
After the 2nd vaccination, the 77-year-old fell ill with a bladder disease, which led to kidney inflammation and ultimately urosepsis. Admitted to hospital (around 3 August) with arrhythmia and thrombosis in the leg.

Medical history

Myocardial infarction in 2013, pulmonary embolism in 2013, deep vein thrombosis in the leg and apoplexy in 2005, paroxysmal atrial fibrillation, congestive dermatosis on the lower leg, chronic constipation with type 2 diabetes mellitus, obstructive sleep apnoea, paralytic ileus (successfully treated).

Autopsy (pathology)

Cause of death: Urosepsis with cardiac decompensation with pre-existing myocardial hypertrophy, arterial hypertension and diabetes mellitus.

Male body with obesity (permagna). Full myocardial hypertrophy (heart weight 1000 g), myocardial scarring after infarction and stent insertion, pronounced arteriosclerosis with coronary sclerosis. Purulent left side pyelonephritis.

Secondary pathohistological examination
The clinically described pyelonephritis and the clinically indicated purulent inflammation of the urinary tract were found. In the prostate there was a histo-morphological severe, purely **lymphocytic inflammation** without detectable purulent abscesses.
Due to the positive spike protein and nucleocapsid detection, a combination of **spike protein-induced tissue damage due to vaccination and viral infection** is evident; or an initially purulent pyelonephritis turned chronic after about 4 weeks and led to corresponding residual findings in the urinary tract tissues. It is currently unclear whether the COVID-19 infection occurred before or after the vaccination and may have been asymptomatic. A combination of vaccination and COVID-19 infection may therefore have contributed to illness and death, with the vaccination probably playing the greater role. However, there were also serious pre-existing conditions that may have caused the death, in particular cardiac damage with massive cardiac hypertrophy and previous myocardial infarctions.
Despite these pre-existing conditions, a connection between the COVID-19 vaccinations and the death is **likely.**

59y / f / 1x Com / 24 **C20**
History of death and vaccination
The 59-year-old died on 21 April 2021 at home in the stairwell.
1st vaccination on 28 March 2021 with Comirnaty ER7812, death 24 days later
Reported COVID-19 disease in January 2021 (2 to 3 months before the COVID-19 vaccination).
Date of death according to daughter's report: After about 5 hours of gardening, she lay down at 9 pm. About half an hour later, severe coughing attacks began, repeated coughing at intervals of about 3 minutes. She asked her husband to call an ambulance. No one answered after dialling the emergency service 112. The husband therefore decided to drive his wife to hospital, but she said she couldn't manage to walk down the stairs. A neighbour then called 112 and got through. After descending one floor, the 59-year-old leant against the wall and slowly slid to the floor. The husband and neighbours provided layman resuscitation until the emergency medical team arrived on the scene. The declared time of death was 11 pm.
The body was confiscated due to the unexplained cause of death and transferred to the forensic medicine department for an autopsy. However, the body was not opened, as a forensic pathologist saw no evidence of any third-party involvement during the by law required post-mortem examination. The public prosecutor subsequently issued a burial certificate. With the support of a lawyer, the relatives obtained a post-mortem examination.

Autopsy (pathology)

Cause of death: bolus event with aspiration, food particles found in various bronchial branches. There were signs of coronary arteriosclerosis and full heart failure with acute decompensation and congestion in the lungs and liver. Vascular thrombi, especially in the pulmonary vessels, could not be detected.

Underlying disease:

- Grade I obesity
- Steatosis hepatis (fatty liver)
- Chronic micro-angiopathy of the skin without thrombi
- Coronary heart disease
- Chronic heart failure and myocardial hypertrophy
- Lipomatosis cordis
- Emphysema of the lungs, possibly as a remnant of a case of COVID-19 pneumonia

Secondary pathohistological examination

The myocardial tissue showed the histo-pathological picture of **myocarditis.**
Together with the immunohistochemical **detection of the spike protein** and the lymphocyte markers (positivity of CD8 lymphocytes and CD3 lymphocytes, negative B cells including plasma cells), the pathogenesis of the myocarditis was almost certainly triggered by the toxic effect of the spike protein of the heart. The lymphocyte markers indicate the early phase of myocarditis with positivity of CD8 lymphocytes and CD3 lymphocytes and negativity of B cells and plasma cells. In addition, questionable spike protein positive endothelial markings and clear markings of the myofibroblasts of the vessel walls and the perivascular inflammatory cells.
Aorta with textural distortion, focal medial dissection and band-like expression of spike protein in myofibroblasts.
In the lungs there is **acute interstitial pneumonia** with hyaline membranes in the alveoli as an indication of a toxic cause (e. g. spike protein or viral RNA). Spike protein expression was detected immunohistochemically in pneumocytes and endothelia of the capillaries and in smaller interstitial blood vessels.
Lymphocytic endothelialitis was conspicuous in the spleen. In addition, spike protein detection in individual lymphocytic cells, periarteriolar and in the red pulp – suggesting the possibility of spike protein toxicity.
Nucleocapsid was negative in all tissues analysed. The spike protein could in principle also originate from a COVID-19 infection, a COVID-19 infection was reported in January 2021, i. e. about 2 months before the COVID-19 vaccination and 3 months before death. However, no nucleocapsid was detectable by immunohistochemistry, which should be present in the same amounts as the spike protein after a viral infection. We therefore assume that the detection of the S1 subunit of the spike protein in the lung and spleen tissue was a consequence of the COVID-19 vaccination and not the reported COVID-19 infection. The pathohistological findings confirm COVID-19 vaccine damage, with severe damage to the heart and lungs adding up.
The death was **almost certainly** caused by the COVID-19 vaccination. Most likely, it was the sole cause.

85y / m / 1x Com / 43 **C21**

History of death and vaccination

The 85-year-old died in hospital on 8 September 2021.
1st vaccination on 27 July 2021 with Comirnaty 1D020A, death 43 days later.
No further vaccination as he suffered a stroke on 20 August (ischaemia in the left middle cerebral artery) and was admitted to hospital on 23 August. He was also diagnosed with acute myeloid leukaemia (AML).

Medical history

Diabetes mellitus type 2

Autopsy (pathology)

Cause of death: heart failure with recurrent myocardial infarction, peripheral pulmonary artery embolism. Cardiac hypertrophy (605 g), pronounced generalised atherosclerosis and coronary sclerosis (RIVA up to 75 %). Myocardial infarction of the anterior wall with involvement of the papillary muscles (3.7 x 2.2 cm) and the posterior wall.
Histology: Partial myocardial fibrosis corresponding to an old, now recurrent infarction. Stretching of the heart valves. Severe chronic, scarred pericarditis. Peripheral pulmonary artery embolisms with evidence of thrombi in the prostatic plexus, most likely the source of the embolism.
Secondary findings: known AML with corresponding bone marrow (60 % blastic cells).

Secondary pathohistological examination

Almost **generalised lymphocytic vasculitis.** Lymphocytic infiltrates in the lungs and prostate. Perivascular lymphocytes in the brain. Non-infarct-related **pericarditis** with pronounced lymphocytic infiltrations. **Pulmonary artery thrombi,** which are rather localised according to the picture of Behçet's syndrome.
The cause of death was probably cardiac failure of a heart previously damaged by infarction with an increase in resistance in the pulmonary circulation with secondary right heart failure.
Due to the clear spike protein expression in the inflammatory cells of the pericarditis and questionable spike expression in the lymphocytic cells of the spleen, a connection between the death and the vaccination is **probably** consistent with a COVID-19 vaccine-induced perimyocarditis.

81y / f / 3x UNKN / 281, 260, 17 **C24**

History of death and vaccination

The 81-year-old woman died on 6 December 2021 after admission to the emergency department following cardiovascular arrest.
1st vaccination on 28 February 2021 with UNKNOWN, death 281 days later
2nd vaccination on 21 March 2021 with UNKNOWN, death 260 days later
3rd vaccination on 19 November 2021 with UNKNOWN, death 17 days later

Admission, intubated and ventilated after she collapsed at home and was initially resuscitated by a layperson. Cardiovascular arrest with known sclerotic cardiomyopathy with high-grade right heart decompensation.
Known pre-existing 'sick sinus syndrome' with chronic atrial fibrillation and right bundle branch block as well as arterial hypertension, bronchial asthma and condition after fracture of the trochanter at the hip joint in July. Condition after taking Pradaxa (Dabigatran – modern anticoagulant as an alternative to Marcumar) for the treatment of atrial fibrillation. This was discontinued due to anaemia.

Autopsy (pathology)
Cause of death: acute myocardial ischaemia. General arteriosclerosis, stenosing coronary sclerosis, acute myocardial ischaemia of the inner layer of the left ventricle, dilatation of all cardiac cavities, pulmonary congestion and oedema, abdominal organ congestion, pleural effusions on both sides, ascites.

Secondary pathohistological examination
Micro-angiopathy predominantly in the myocardium with **lymphocytic peri- and myocarditis. Lymphocytic infiltrates in the lungs** and **onion-skin-like arteriolitis in the spleen.** With regard to the vascular changes in the myocardium, similar changes in the cerebral vessels may also have been present. No specimens are available.
There was a paraffin-embedded tissue sample from the spleen. We were able to carry out immunohistochemical analysis of the spike protein. Cytoplasmic and perinuclear positivity of individual lymphoid cells were found. Endothelium and exfoliated endothelia were also positive. No other tissue samples were available for additional immunohistochemical analysis. The epi-myocarditis in itself already speaks in favour of a causal connection with the triple COVID-19 vaccination. This connection is confirmed by the positive detection of spike protein in vascular endothelia and lymphoid cells of the spleen.
There is **almost certainly** a connection between the COVID-19 vaccinations and death.

C28

63y / m / 1x Com / 36
History of death and vaccination
The 63-year-old died on 26 February 2022.
1st vaccination on 21 January 2022 with Comirnaty FH0161, death 36 days later

Autopsy (pathology)
Cause of death: acute myocardial infarction in the posterior wall of the left ventricle with pre-existing general atherosclerosis and stenosing coronary sclerosis.
Myocardial callosities in the left ventricle, lymphocytic vasculitis of the right side coronary artery in the histology, hypertrophy of the left and right ventricle, dilatation of all cardiac cavities, acute pulmonary congestion, congestion of the parenchymal abdominal organs, fatty liver and fatty liver hepatitis.

Histology: Myocardium of the left ventricle with callosities and acute myocardial infarction. Pronounced coronary sclerosis and lymphocytic arteritis of the arteria coronaria dextra and the vasa vasorum. Fatty liver and fatty liver hepatitis – both nutritive-toxic genesis and non-alcoholic steatohepatitis possible.

Secondary pathohistological examination
Typical vaccine-associated changes were found in several organs: **Lymphocytic infiltrates in the lungs.** In the spleen, onion-skin like arteritis and material of uncertain origin. Typical endothelialitis of small vessels also in the brain (striatum) with haemosiderosis.
Pre-existing atherosclerosis, coronary sclerosis and extensive myocardial callosities. However, acute media dissection and pericoronitis, **amyloid-like cushion formations** in small arterioles. Isolated acute myocardial necrosis. In the case of pre-existing atherosclerosis and old heart attacks, the final heart failure is probably caused by the additional fresh vascular changes after the COVID-19 vaccination. Spike protein markings were visible immunohistochemically in the vessel wall of the coronary artery in the area of the dissection.
A connection between the death and the previous COVID-19 vaccination is **probable.**

86y / f / 2x Com / 344, 302 **C29**
History of death and vaccination
The 86-year-old woman considered herself to be quite fit for her age until the vaccinations. Her relatives confirmed this. Shortly after the vaccinations, the sequence of illnesses leading to death described below set in. Death on 14 December 2021.
1st vaccination on 4 January 2021 with Comirnaty, batch number unknown, death 344 days later
2nd vaccination on 15 February 2021 with Comirnaty, batch number unknown, death 302 days later
In March 2021, a moderately differentiated adenocarcinoma was removed, sigmoid diverticulosis. The planned hemicolectomy in April 2021 was not performed as the colon mucosa was normal in the colonoscopy.
In May 2021, a thrombosis in the foot was diagnosed without evidence of thrombosis in the upper half of the body.
In June 2021, exertional dyspnoea with general weakness and bronchitis/alveolitis was diagnosed. In addition, moderate mitral valve insufficiency and a complete left bundle branch block.
In October 2021, the patient was hospitalised with pulmonary artery embolism with infarct pneumonia and several bleeding ulcers in the duodenum. Echocardiography diagnosed hypertrophic heart disease with normal left ventricular pump function. On admission, the 86-year-old was in a reduced general condition.
In November 2021, a complicated bladder infection with E. coli and an uncertain mass in the bladder with recurrent bleeding were diagnosed with simultaneous Apixaban anticoagulation therapy following the pulmonary embolism in the previ-

ous month. In December, the 86-year-old woman was hospitalised as a multimorbid patient until her death on 14 December 2021.

Autopsy (forensic medicine)
Petite female corpse: 155 cm, 49 kg.
Cause of death: respiratory failure due to advanced pneumonia. The bladder mucosa was thickened due to chronic complicated cystitis, not tumorous, probably due to chronic urinary retention. Large bowel diverticulum, no tumour visible.

Secondary pathohistological examination
A number of typical vaccine-associated vascular wall changes were found, in particular **endothelialitis, media necrosis of arteries, amyloid deposits** in vascular walls and an older media haemorrhage in medium-sized cerebral vessels. In the spleen, hyaline wall swelling was found in arterioles, onion skin phenomenon and massive haemorrhages in vessel wall damage.
Immunohistochemically, weak spike protein positivity was found in the myocytes of the heart and in the brain. Since the last coronavirus vaccination took place 302 days before death, it is also conceivable that additional spike protein exposure due to a COVID-19 infection occurred between the last vaccination and death. This could explain the weak positive immunohistochemical nucleocapsid positivity in the myocytes of the heart.
The main cause of death was inflammatory infiltrates in the heart muscle with pronounced inflammation of the pericardium. The last direct cause of death was probably the onset of granulocytic pneumonia. No foreign material was found in any of the organs.
The COVID-19 vaccination **almost certainly** played a decisive role in the pathogenesis leading to death.

C30

39y / m / 3x Com / 357, 336, 56
History of death and vaccination
The 39-year-old died suddenly and unexpectedly on 10 January 2021.
1st vaccination on 18 January 2021 with Comirnaty EJ6769, death 357 days later
2nd vaccination on 8 February 2021 with Comirnaty EJ6134, death 336 days later
3rd vaccination on 15 November 2021 with Comirnaty SH0161, death 56 days later
The first 2 vaccinations were administered by a family doctor, the 3rd vaccination in a vaccination centre. He was always sickly after the vaccinations (at least twice) with fever and exhaustion.
No serious previous illnesses. According to reports from his sister, he was happily married, father of three children aged 3, 5 and 8, managing director and owner of a company with over 50 employees, also maintained his friendships and managed to successfully realise his life goals with ease. In recent months, he occasionally complained of headaches and sometimes tension in his neck after strenuous sporting activities (football, tennis, mountain biking). As a small child he had febrile convulsions.

Autopsy (pathology)
Cause of death: cerebral infarction.
- Softening of the right temporal lobe – macroscopic infarction
- Inflammation of the trachea and oesophagus
- Congestion of blood in internal organs
- Pulmonary oedema
- Increased fragility of the lungs

Secondary pathohistological examination
Pronounced **vascular changes** such as media necrosis, fragmentation, perivasculitis and endothelialitis as well as hyaline wall deposits, probably amyloid. The vessel walls of the spleen showed an onion skin pattern.
Also found in the spleen, liver and myocardium were partly exposed, partly vacuolar **brownish, granular, rod-shaped deposits** of unknown origin.
Lymphocytic infiltrates were found in the lungs and in the thyroid gland with the appearance of Hashimoto's **thyroiditis.** Minor lymphocytic **myocarditis,** predominantly on the right.
Vascular changes, especially in the brain, with fragmentation of lymphocytic inflammation and focal haemosiderosis. These changes are consistent with the autopsy findings of a **cerebral infarction.**
A connection between the death and the previous triple COVID-19 vaccination is **almost certainly** given, especially since no other serious organ changes were found that could point to an alternative cause of death. This is confirmed by the exquisitely positive spike protein detection in the damaged organ structures, especially the aorta.

56y / m / 1x UNKN, 1x Com / 45, 20 **C31**
History of death and vaccination
The 56-year-old died on 13 February 2022.
1st vaccination on 30 December 2021 with UNKNOWN, death 45 days later
2nd vaccination on 24 January 2022 with Comirnaty (batch number cannot be taken from the printout of the EU digital COVID certificate), death 20 days later
Since 7 February 2022 malaise, pallor and weakness. On 12 February 2022 emergency admission with acute coronary syndrome. ST elevation, myocardial infarction. Emergency cardiac catheterisation with wire recanalisation and thrombaspiration of the proximal right coronary artery, stent placement in the medial and distal right coronary artery and direct stent placement in the proximal right coronary artery. Deterioration (confusion, cardiorespiratory decompensation). Transoesophageal echocardiography shows infarct-related septal rupture and inferobasal aneurysm formation. Oxygenation through ECMO therapy. Around midnight cardiorespiratory deterioration, refractory ventricular fibrillation and death. Transoesophageal echocardiography to clarify the cause revealed free aortic valve insufficiency and a dissection of the aorta.

Autopsy (pathology)
Cause of death: Cardiogenic shock as a result of aortic dissection in the ascending part (Stanford type A) with pericardial tamponade. This was preceded by an acute myocardial infarction with ST elevation and a haemodynamically critical ventricular septum defect.
Slightly obese (BMI 25.7) male corpse. Signs of underlying disease include generalised atherosclerosis with high-grade coronary sclerosis (stent in the main branch of the right coronary artery) in right-sided supply type. Diffuse fibrosis zones in the left myocardium as a feature of chronic ischaemic heart disease. Hypertensive heart disease with pronounced left ventricular hypertrophy, signs of pulmonary hypertension with severely dilated right ventricle, signs of chronic hepatic and splenic congestion. Pulmonary emphysema, anthracosis.
Minor reactive lymphadenopathy in the area of the left axilla.
The post-mortem examiner reported this case to the Paul-Ehrlich-Institut as a possible suspected case of vaccination complication in accordance with the Infection Protection Act.

Secondary pathohistological examination
The histological organ and tissue changes are generally compatible with vaccine-associated damage. The detection of spike proteins in the wall of coronary arteries in the presence of pre-existing atherosclerosis and pronounced dissection with an inflammatory reaction suggests that the myocardial infarction that was undoubtedly present was already caused by the **spike protein-induced coronary artery lesions.**
The myocardial infarction was treated clinically and survived. The immediate cause of death was an **aortic dissection with rupture** and haemorrhage, as already established at the initial autopsy. The significant inflammatory reaction in the dissection area would not be compatible with idiopathic microcystic media necrosis, nor with atherosclerotic vascular damage.The pattern of damage to the aorta and coronary artery corresponds to changes following intoxication (e.g. lathyrism). In fact, the toxic spike protein, which is COVID-19 vaccine-induced, could be detected selectively in damaged sections of the aorta with dissection and rupture.
The fatal haemorrhage after aortic rupture must therefore be clearly classified as a consequence of vaccination. The two COVID-19 vaccinations and the death are therefore **almost certainly** related.

C34

79y / m / 2x Com / 144, 108
History of death and vaccination
The 79-year-old died on 30 October 2021 after 6 days in hospital, to which he had been admitted due to recurrent falls.
1st vaccination on 8 June 2021 with Comirnaty 1D018A, death 144 days later
2nd vaccination on 14 July 2021 with Comirnaty 1E029A, death 108 days later
According to the son-in-law, the 79-year-old had survived the first vaccination without any problems. However, two weeks after the second vaccination in July 2021,

trembling of hands and memory impairment occurred. At the end of September, beginning of October, he fell 4 times within 2 weeks "as if struck by lightning", without any defence reaction (always on the back of his head). In mid-October, he then started to see things that weren't there. "He kept tearing his clothes off because he was supposedly so hot."

His last stay in hospital was from 24 October 2021 to the day of his death, 30 October. He was admitted to hospital in an emergency due to recurrent falls, most recently 10 days earlier (13 October) on the back of his head with an occipital laceration, which was surgically treated. In the two weeks prior to this, the tendency to fall had worsened considerably, accompanied by changes in character and a deterioration in general health. Apparently, the 79-year-old had been lying down for days and had suffered a sacral decubitus ulcer.

On admission, he was disorientated, somnolent with tremor and reduced vigilance. Imaging excluded sinus thrombosis, basilar artery thrombosis or brain ischaemia. Generalised brain atrophy with moderate micro-angiopathic changes on MRI.

Cheyne-Stokes respiration was reported three days before death. He developed fever and further deterioration of the general condition. Empirical treatment for meningitis/encephalitis with Ceftriaxone, Ampicillin and Acyclovir was administered. The lumbar puncture revealed only "slight signs of barrier dysfunction". Blood and urine cultures remained sterile. Deceased on 30 October 2021 in the evening.

- ECG: sinus rhythm, over-twisted left type, left anterior hemiblock
- SARS-CoV-2 PCR: negative 2 times
- Blood count: macrocytic anaemia (Hb 6.0 mmol/L, MCV 110 fL, erythrocytes 3.00 Tpt/L)
- Signs of inflammation (leucocytes and CRP elevated)
- Electrolyte imbalance (hypernatraemia, hypocalcaemia, creatinine and urea elevated, uric acid elevated)

Autopsy (pathology)

Causes of death: Heart failure with pre-existing atherosclerosis and COVID-19 infection with respiratory insufficiency (SARS-CoV-2 PCR from lung swab negative). The autopsy revealed decompensated cor pulmonale, abscessing hypostatic pneumonia with pre-existing chronic emphysema bronchitis. S. aureus and C. albicans in the lung smear.

Infected sacral decubitus with blackish discolouration. Pressure ulcer on the left heel. Caries profunda with cutaneous fistula. Generalised osteoporosis, beam bladder with prostatic hyperplasia. Colonic diverticulosis with diverticulitis. Recurrent urinary tract infections.

Secondary pathohistological examination

There are definite changes in small and larger blood vessels in the heart muscle and in capillaries in the brain, which indicate vaccine damage.

Abscessed herd pneumonia must be regarded as the immediate **cause of death,** although the very pronounced, obviously **COVID-19 vaccine-induced organ damage**

in the heart, blood vessels and brain made a significant contribution to the death. This is confirmed by the focal spike protein expression in myofibroblast cells of the outer coronary artery wall.
A connection between the death and the COVID-19 vaccinations that had taken place was therefore considered **probable.**

C42

84y / f / 1x Johnson, 1x UNKN / 259, 17-33

History of death and vaccination

On 23 February 2022, the 84-year-old woman was found dead at home, two weeks after leaving the hospital where she had been admitted due to facial shingles. A digital vaccination certificate was found on her smartphone:
1st vaccination on 9 June 2021 with Johnson, batch number unknown – however, the son doubts the authenticity as the woman did not actually want to be vaccinated
2nd vaccination with UNKNOWN, potential vaccination period: 22 January to 7 February 2022 (hospitalisation)
In February, the 84-year-old woman had facial shingles and was hospitalised. There she was temporarily very confused and said that she had received an injection as well as tablets. After 10 days in hospital in isolation, she tested positive for COVID-19 and was completely asymptomatic. The hospital report makes no mention of a COVID-19 vaccination, but relatives suspect that she was nevertheless vaccinated. After her discharge, the residual findings of the zoster infection gradually improved and she became stronger again.

Autopsy (pathology)

Cause of death: Cardiac failure due to pericardial tamponade caused by haemorrhagic pericardial effusion.
Origin of the pericardial haemorrhage somewhat unclear. No myocardial rupture, no major endothelial lesion of the aorta. Adventitia of the ascending and descending aorta is diffusely haemorrhaged over a distance of approx. 25 cm from the aortic valve. Furthermore, deep leg vein thrombosis over 10 cm. No pulmonary embolism detectable.

Secondary pathohistological examination

The immunohistochemical detection of the **spike protein in the vessel wall of the aorta** in both aortic specimens with negative immunohistochemistry for the nucleocapsid suggests that one or more COVID-19 vaccinations have taken place.
Based on the findings on the aorta, it must be assumed that there was a dissection of the aorta with macroscopically visible haemorrhage into the aortic wall as well as spreading and haemorrhage into the pericardium at autopsy. The cause of the **aortic dissection** is obviously a considerable inflammation in the intima area without significant atheromatous beds as well as a dissection in the deep medial area with media necrosis and incipient inflammatory infiltration. Such lesions of the large vessels are typically found after COVID-19 vaccinations, where the spike protein apparently destroys elastic layers.

This causal link is supported by immunohistological positivity of the spike protein in the lesion zones of the aorta. The causal link between one or more COVID-19 vaccinations and the fatal haemorrhage into the aortic wall and pericardium is therefore **almost certainly** established.

29y / m / 2x Com / 97, 67 **C46**

History of death and vaccination

The previously healthy 29-year-old died suddenly and unexpectedly on 5 February 2022 while training in a gym.
1st vaccination on 31 October 2021 with Comirnaty FF2834, death 97 days later
2nd vaccination on 30 November 2021 with Comirnaty FK6303, death 67 days later

Autopsy (pathology)

Cause of death: Pronounced extensive haemorrhages in the lungs intra-alveolar. One section shows a large lymphocytic infiltrate. Image consistent with Goodpasture syndrome.

Secondary pathohistological examination

Extensive COVID-19 vaccine-typical **vascular damage with cystic media necrosis** was found in the **aorta and arteries. Endothelialitis** was also found in smaller vessels of the brain, some of which were obliterating. The myocardial scars in the absence of arteriosclerosis/coronary sclerosis are likely to be a few months old and may already be **myocarditis scars** and thus the result of vaccination (the 1st COVID-19 vaccination took place a little more than 3 months before the sudden and unexpected death; this was followed by the 2nd vaccination a little more than 2 months before death).
The immediate cause of death was confirmed as acute, extensive, fresh **alveolar haemorrhages.**
Since only histological sections were available, no specimens were available to make further sections and no further immunohistochemical examinations could be carried out. In particular, the immunohistochemical tests for the spike protein would be of interest to confirm whether the COVID-19 vaccinations that took place led to the tissue and vascular damage described.
However, the pathohisto-morphological picture of the inflammatory vascular changes in particular, corresponds to that which the investigating pathologists Burkhardt and Lang repeatedly saw in people who died after COVID-19 vaccinations.
Even independently of immunohistochemical spike detection, the COVID-19 vaccine-typical vascular lesions (which were also found in the lungs), constitute a probability for a connection between the death and the vaccinations **bordering** on **certainty.**

C47

51y / m / 2x Com, 1x Mod / 262, 220, 40

History of death and vaccination

On the morning of 23 January 2022, the 51-year-old collapsed, was still responsive but already unconscious when the emergency physician arrived; resuscitation attempts were unsuccessful. No known previous illnesses.

1st vaccination on 6 May 2021 with Comirnaty ET3045, death 262 days later
2nd vaccination on 17 June 2021 with Comirnaty 1D017A, death 220 days later
3rd vaccination on 14 December 2021 with Moderna 042G21A, death 40 days later
On the evening of October 2021, pain occurred in the right shoulder, which increasingly moved towards the thoracic vertebrae. After the "booster vaccination" in December, cardiac constriction and shortness of breath occurred. On 17 January 2022 the doctor prescribed physiotherapy.

Autopsy (forensic medicine)

Cause of death: Sudden cardiac arrhythmia with considerable calcification of the coronary arteries in a natural way.

Main findings: Severe calcification of the coronary arteries with subtotal narrowing of the descending branch of the left coronary artery due to lemon peel looking deposits and partially organised clot material. In the past, this coronary artery calcification had already led to myocardial cell destruction in the form of small myocardial infarctions, which appeared as small areas of scarring within the musculature. The pain between the shoulder blades reported in the case history can be interpreted as angina pectoris pain in view of the autopsy findings.

Secondary pathohistological examination

Only moderate general atherosclerosis, but pronounced, calcifying **atheromatous coronary sclerosis with wall dissection and perivasculitis.** Extensive old myocardial scars, next to necrotic acute foci of necrosis. Peripheral **pulmonary embolisms** due to particle deposits and small pulmonary infarction. Death probably due to recurrent myocardial infarctions in inflammatory coronary artery lesions and peripheral pulmonary infarctions and embolisms. As it has often been the case in people who died after COVID-19 vaccinations, partly exposed, partly **vacuolar, black-brown, crystalline particles** were found in the **pancreas, lungs and heart.**

The vascular inflammatory lymphocytic manifestations of the coronary arteries show the now familiar pathohistological picture of COVID-19 vaccine-induced vascular inflammation. However, immunohistochemical spike detection was unsuccessful in heart sections. In the cerebrum, immunohisto-chemically weak spike protein markings of endothelial cells of small vessels were found. In the lungs there were isolated cytoplasmic granular spike protein markings.

Signs of vasculitis were found in the brain area with older micro haemorrhages (haemosiderosis).

A connection between the death and the COVID-19 vaccination seems **very likely.**

C49

56y / m / 3x Mod / 336, 296, 104
History of death and vaccination
1st vaccination on 15 April 2021 with Moderna 3001651, death 336 days later
2nd vaccination on 25 May 2021 with Moderna 3002334, death 296 days later
3rd vaccination on 3 December 2021 with Moderna 3005690, death 104 days later
According to the wife's reports, a 'vaccination arm' appeared after the 1st vaccination, which also hurt during sleep. After the 2nd vaccination, she noticed increasing pallor, also in photos, and he "looked ill". After the summer holiday, he was very unwell and went to the doctor on 6 September, where he was diagnosed with high blood pressure and treated with antihypertensives:

- BiPreterax (ACE inhibitor)
- Viacorind (Perindopril, Amlodipine and Indapamide)
- Lercanidipine-Omniapharm

Long-term blood pressure measurements were made with peak systolic around 180 mmHg. Gradual improvement and cessation. The patient was a heavy smoker and was therefore particularly afraid of COVID-19.
On the day of death (17 March 2022) he suddenly had chest pain in the morning. He later visited the doctor (for treatment of a hand injury). At 3:20 pm, the wife found her husband on the terrace bench with his upper body hanging over the back of the bench to the left, head blue, hands blue. Resuscitation attempts were unsuccessful.

Post-mortem examination (forensic medicine)
"Type of death natural causes."
Cause of death: The autopsy revealed a ruptured atheroma bed in the wrap-around branch of the left coronary artery. Macroscopically, the lumen was almost occluded, or at least severely narrowed. The picture was that of an acute myocardial infarction.

Secondary pathohistological examination
The coronary artery changes make an acute infarction plausible, but the image of a classic myocardial infarction was not found in the myocardial tissue. If the coronary occlusion was the cause of death, this led to a rapid death (immediate cardiac death) without morphologically visible, intravital ischaemic damage in the myocardial tissue. **Inflammation of an inner vessel wall** led to 'cushion formation' inwards with narrowing of the vessel lumen. In addition, the risk of thrombus formation increased in inflamed vessels. The now frequently described 'sudden adult death' syndrome can be triggered by such an acute occlusion of a coronary vessel.
We were able to see lymphocytic inflammation typical of COVID-19 vaccination in the coronary vessels, and the immunohistochemical detection of the spike protein in the myofibroblasts of the coronary artery wall and its branches speaks in favour of vaccine-toxic vascular damage at a vital site.
The death is therefore **almost certainly** related to the 3 COVID-19 vaccinations that took place.

C56

85y / m / 1x Com / 59

History of death and vaccination

The 85-year-old died on the night of 18 October 2021 in a university hospital in the presence of his son.

1st vaccination on 20 August 2021 with Comirnaty SCKX7, death 59 days later

The 85-year-old had cataracts and wanted to have eye surgery at the beginning of September 2021. During a visit to his family doctor on 20 August 2021 for pre-operative examinations, she urged him to accept a COVID-19 vaccination, as otherwise eye surgery would not be possible.

Seven days after the vaccination (on 27 August), he was unable to move at night and experienced severe pain. The following day, the emergency doctor diagnosed a urinary tract infection with urinary retention and suspected renal colic. Treatment with strong painkillers and an antibiotic brought relief.

On 30 August 2021: Hospital: there he was put on laxatives, he tripped and fell to the floor twice.

On 8 September 2021: Hospitalisation for spinal surgery. High inflammatory parameters and signs of kidney failure; suspected plasmacytoma.

On 24 September 2021: University hospital. No plasmocytoma diagnosed, kidney biopsy.

On 2 October 2021: Dialysis. Under dialysis, deterioration of general condition with water retention and increasing confusion. Additional pneumonia. Diagnosis of CMV virus.

Senior physician obtained consent from relatives for publication of the case as a COVID-19 vaccination episode. However, the publication was never submitted.

Medical history

The 85-year-old had been suffering from polymyalgia rheumatica for years, had already had three strokes (once in 1997 and twice in 2011), received a pacemaker in 2016 and was treated in 2021 for vasoconstriction in his legs. An operation was not performed due to severe heart failure. In his younger years, he had been severely affected by shingles.

Autopsy (pathology)

The autopsy was started, but the body was confiscated by order of the public prosecutor's office and transferred to the Institute of Forensic Medicine.

Autopsy (Institute of Forensic Medicine)

An autopsy report is not available.

Secondary pathohistological examination

There were clear, typically COVID-19 vaccine-associated tissue changes: In the heart there was **lymphocytic myocarditis** with myocardial fibre destruction consistent with massive myocarditis, practically no granulocytes (as would be the case with an infarction). In the heart muscle, we were able to detect the **spike protein** by immunohistochemistry, which the body cells are induced to produce by the COVID-19 vaccinations. Spike protein positivity was found in the endothelia, vessel walls and

myofibroblasts in the pericardial fatty tissue. Spike protein positivity was also found in the myocardial fibres, particularly in scar fields with signs of necrobiosis. Microvasculitis was found in the brain with residual haemorrhages in the vessel wall. Spike protein typical inflammatory vascular changes were also found in the lungs. Typical vacuolar, **brownish crystalline, rod- and fan-shaped non-localised materials** were found in the pancreas in particular. Such material deposits are repeatedly found in people who have died after COVID-19 vaccination. The composition and origin of these material deposits is unknown. It is also not known whether they are of pathogenetic significance or may even have been involved in the death process.
The **spike protein expression** in the **testicles** is irrelevant for the disease and death, but is remarkable for the gain in knowledge about the pathophysiological effects of COVID-19 vaccinations, also with regard to a possible reduction in fertility.
In the spleen, a vascular wall loosening, consistent with an **'onion skin pattern'** was found, which is also typical for spleen findings in people who died after COVID-19 vaccination. Remarkable is also the atrophy of the spleen and lymph nodes consistent with a lack of stimulation (that one would have expected from a vaccination).
The final cause of death was probably abscessing pneumonia. However, the findings show that the COVID-19 vaccination had led to inflammatory damage, especially to the vascular walls throughout the body, and was therefore a decisive factor in the course of the disease.
A connection between the COVID-19 vaccination and death is therefore **probable.**

93y / f / 3x Com / 305, 263, 39 **C58**

History of death and vaccination

The 93-year-old woman died in hospital on 27 February 2022.
1st vaccination on 28 April 2021 with Comirnaty EX3510, death 305 days later
2nd vaccination on 9 June 2021 with Comirnaty FA5833, death 263 days later
3rd vaccination approx. on 19 January 2022 with Comirnaty 1F1027A, death 39 days later
The 93-year-old was still remarkably fit for her age. She lived independently and was able to walk well (1 – 2 hours of leisurely walking without a rollator walker was possible). Had level 1 care (= lowest care grade in German health system) with cleaning assistance as of the year 2020. Declining cognitive performance in summer 2021. First massive physical collapse in mid-October 2021 with admission to hospital in an ambulance. Since then, insulin injections, blood glucose derailments, cramps, chronic calcifying pancreatitis. Subsequently 6 hospital stays in 6 different hospitals until death on 27 February 2022.
Acute gallbladder inflammation in December 2021. From 3rd January 2022 she had been hospitalised due to a depressive episode. Until two days before her death, she was quarantined in a hospital room with fellow patients due to a positive COVID-19 test. During these 20 days in quarantine, she had not shown any COVID-19 symptoms but, according to her daughter, had deteriorated mentally and cognitively.

On 27 February, the nursing staff noticed an acute deterioration in her general condition. She was transferred to a university hospital with snap breathing and abdominal problems. Cardiovascular arrest on admission to the university hospital. No resuscitation was carried out due to the patient's instructions in her living will.

Medical history
Atrial fibrillation with intake of blood thinners. Allergies to bee and wasp stings.

Autopsy (forensic medicine)
Cause of death: Peritonitis, probably as a result of renewed gallbladder inflammation, pneumonia (with positive SARS-CoV-2 test). However, due to the severity of the peritonitis, the pneumonia was probably of secondary importance.
High-grade coronary arteriosclerosis, high-grade general arterio-arteriolosclerosis. Pulmonary arteriosclerosis.
Furthermore: Nodular altered thyroid gland, atrophy of the pancreas, dilatation of the duct and stones. Benign tumour of the meninges (meningioma).

Secondary pathohistological examination
Chronic, partially abscessing cholecystitis and pericholecystitis. Diffuse alveolar damage with possible aspiration. Conspicuous lymphocytic component.
Lymphocytic **vasculitis of small vessels** in the **cerebrum.** Non-localised particles in hepatocytes of the liver. **Media necrosis of the coronary arteries** with inflammation and perivasculitis, focally pronounced with stenosis. Immunohistochemistry revealed the expression of the spike protein in the myocardial tissue in the absence of the nucleocapsid. The cause of death was acute heart failure due to coronary artery lesions, which may have been caused by spike protein toxicity.
A connection between the death and the COVID-19 vaccinations that took place is **probable.** This is supported by the spike protein detection, especially in the vessel walls.

C60

72y / f / 3x Com / 271, 234, 19
History of death and vaccination
The 72-year-old died on 23 January 2022 in the intensive care unit of a hospital.
1st vaccination on 27 April 2021 with Comirnaty EX3599, death 271 days later
2nd vaccination on 3 June 2021 with Comirnaty 1D016A, death 234 days later
3rd vaccination on 4 January 2022 with Comirnaty ACB4694, death 19 days later
According to her son, the 72-year-old woman was fit and could still walk with her son. She had already complained of dizziness and headaches after the 1st vaccination. Medical examinations were inconclusive. After the 3rd vaccination 4 of January, she suffered a stroke on 15 January, during which she fell into a coma from which she never woke up. She was intubated in the intensive care unit and died there on 23 January 2022.

Autopsy (forensic medicine)
According to the death certificate, death on 23 January 2022 at 5:12 pm due to "respiratory insufficiency" as a result of an increase in intracranial pressure with incarceration of brain tissue caused by an intracerebral haemorrhage.
At autopsy, fresh haemorrhages were found above and below the meninges in the area of the cerebellum and in the cerebellar tissue.
Cause of death: Extensive cerebellar haemorrhage. Localisation characteristic of a haemorrhage caused by high blood pressure.

Secondary pathohistological examination
Some tissue changes typically occurring after COVID-19 vaccinations were found: In the cerebrum, microvascular changes with lymphocytic inflammation and signs of micro-haemorrhages were found in several sections. In the splenic arterioles, there was loosening of the vascular wall consistent with an onion-skin phenomenon, as is typically seen after COVID-19 vaccinations. In addition, deposits of **amyloid-like hyaline material** were found in the vessel walls.
The immediate cause of death was obviously the intra **cerebral haemorrhages** in the cerebellum described by the forensic pathologist who performed the autopsy, traces of which could only be identified in the cerebrum in the second examination. In view of the cerebral vascular changes found, these may have been induced by the COVID-19 vaccinations.
This interpretation is supported by the **positive spike protein detection in endothelia** and vessel walls in the heart and spleen as well as occasionally in the brain. It is also supported by the detection of non-cellular, proteinaceous amyloid-like material in the vessel walls.
A connection between the death and the COVID-19 vaccination is therefore **probable.**

74y / f / 1x Astra, 1x Com / 130, 83 **C61**
History of death and vaccination
Since July 2021 progressive dementia, dysphagia, tetraspasticity and myoclonus of the extremities. Died on 14 November 2021 under palliative morphine treatment at the age of 74.
1st vaccination on 7 July 2021 with Astra Zeneca ABW3644, death 130 days later
2nd vaccination on 23 August 2021 with Comirnaty 1D020A, death 83 days later

Medical history
- Suspicion of Creutzfeld-Jakob disease
- Restless legs syndrome
- Stage III lymphoedema of all extremities
- Diabetes mellitus type 2
- Hypothyroidism
- Allergic bronchial asthma
- Cardiac insufficiency

Autopsy (neuropathology)
Brain with signs of spongiform encephalopathy and immunohistochemical positivity of pathological prion proteins consistent with Creutzfeld-Jakob disease (also a reliable diagnosis according to WHO criteria). MM/MV 1 + 2c subtype.

Secondary pathohistological examination
In agreement with the diagnosis of the Neuropathological Institute of the University of Hamburg, clear positivity of neuronal cells on presentation of the prions (foreign sections). In addition, minimal lymphocytic vasculitis and inflammation of the soft meninges in the sections stained here. Sporadic visualisation of spike protein in endothelia and inflammatory cells with negative reaction for nucleocapsid.
A damaging effect of the COVID-19 vaccinations on the brain is **probable.**
A connection with the undoubtedly existing prion disease is possible. There are hypothetical indications of this in the scientific literature, but there is still a lack of experimental scientific evidence.

C62

56y / m / 2x Com / 140, 92
Death and vaccination history
1st vaccination on 5 September 2021 with Comirnaty SCRP9, death 140 days later
2nd vaccination on 23 October 2021 with Comirnaty 1F034A, death 92 days later
The man died on 23 January 2022.

Autopsy (pathology)
Cause of death: Ventricular rupture of the left posterior wall with pericardial tamponade. Fresh, adherent, occlusive thrombus of the posterior interventricular ramus (RIVP). Pre-existing coronary arteriosclerosis with moderate to severe arteriosclerosis. Moderate cardiac hypertrophy on the left, mild on the right. Heart weight 555 g. Multiple patchy, disseminated, fibrous myocardial scars. In the posterior interventricular ramus evidence of an adherent, occlusive thrombus with consecutive ischaemia and rupture of the left posterior wall.
"Due to the pronounced cardiac pre-damage, based on arterial vascular disease, there is no pathological link between the COVID-19 vaccination and the onset of death."

Secondary pathohistological examination
The final posterior wall rupture with fatal pericardial tamponade could certainly be explained by recurrent myocardial infarction with acute necrotic push at the posterior wall. The pre-existing, resorbed older myocardial infarcts in this area could be **necrosis due to spike protein toxins** induced by the vaccinations 92 and 140 days before death. The immunohistochemical positivity of spike protein in the myocardium and in the coronary arteries supports the hypothesis that these older infarctions are the consequences of the COVID-19 vaccinations.
A causal link between the deaths and the two COVID-19 vaccinations that took place therefore seems **very likely.**

C66

48y / m / 2x Com / 191, 172

History of death and vaccination

The 48-year-old died suddenly and unexpectedly on 12 June 2022 on a park bench after previous sporting activities.

1st vaccination on 3 December 2021 with Comirnaty, batch number unknown, death 191 days later

2nd vaccination on 22 December 2021 with Comirnaty, batch number unknown, death 172 days later

Unfortunately, the batch numbers of the BioNTech Comirnaty doses vaccinated cannot be found in the "EU Digital COVID Certificates".

The 48-year-old actually wanted to help out as a ski instructor at the local ski school, which was also the reason for the vaccination. A few days after the 2nd vaccination, he developed a high temperature. Since the 2nd vaccination, he also repeatedly reported to his best friend that he felt unwell, both mentally and physically. On the day of his death in mid-June (12 June 2022), he rode his e-bike up a nearby mountain and then took his Vespa to the windsurfing club. After surfing and taking a break on the sunbathing lawn, he felt nauseous and needed to throw up. Went to the toilet. Then immediately sat down on a bench. Sudden outbreak of sweat and gasping. Sank to the side, dead. Resuscitation attempts from 6 pm to 7:30 pm were unsuccessful.

Medical police autopsy (Austria)

No autopsy report available.

Secondary pathohistological examination

Severe vascular changes, massive **mesaortitis and coronary arteritis** were found. In addition, a massive, left-accentuated multifocal confluent **myocarditis.**

Spike protein was also detected immunohistochemically in the patho-histologically correspondingly damaged tissues of the heart, coronary arteries and aorta. With a **high degree of certainty,** the death was the result of the COVID-19 vaccinations.

C71

21y / m / 2x Mod / 95, 53

History of death and vaccination

The 21-year-old was found dead in bed in the morning of 4 August 2021. Resuscitation was no longer possible.

1st vaccination on 1 May 2021 with Moderna 3001651, death 95 days later

2nd vaccination on 12 June 2021 with Moderna 3002620, death 53 days later

In mid-July (11th of July), the 21-year-old suffered from a severe cough. The doctor prescribed cough syrup on 15 July, COVID-19 and whooping cough tests were both negative. Cough calmed down again, but increasing fatigue and tiredness.

Previously in excellent health, high school diploma, dance course, driving licence, second best in the guild examination as an electrician. Involved in the fire brigade, where he was a certified G26 respirator wearer, tractor driver and enjoyed working in the fields with his grandad.

Autopsy (forensic medicine)
Cause of death: still unclear. 175 cm tall, 129 kg male corpse in good general condition. Discolouration of the heart muscles of the cardiac septum, but no clear pathological findings, heart weight 540 g.
Spleen weight 340 g, approx. 0.5 cm large focus on the spleen (so-called secondary spleen).
Patchy haemorrhages in the scalp and under the soft meninges (to a small extent).
Thyroid gland haemostasis.
Findings consistent with an upper influence congestion due to cardiac insufficiency.
Toxicology: alcohol 0.01 per mille, narcotics and drug screening without findings.

The investigation by the public prosecutor's office against unknown person was discontinued in accordance with § 170 paragraph 2 StPO (German Code of Criminal Procedure).

Secondary pathohistological examination
Minimal vascular changes were found, which could possibly be the result of COVID-19 vaccination. The **brownish crystalline particle deposits,** some of which are selectively attached to vessels in the heart and brain, are conspicuous. This material was also found in the liver and massively in the pancreas (as we have often found in pancreatic tissue after COVID-19 vaccinations).
The partly exposed, partly vacuolar, non-local/organic, crystalline particles are a common finding in the analysed autopsy material of people who died after COVID-19 vaccination.
An ultimate cause of death could not be determined. However, a connection with the COVID-19 vaccinations that took place is **probable.**

C72

24y / m / 1x Jan, 1x Com / 177, 56
History of death and vaccination
The 24-year-old was found dead in a locked toilet at the main train train station in Mannheim (Germany), where he had previously arrived on an "Intercity Express". After one and a half hours of unsuccessful resuscitation, he was pronounced dead at the University Hospital.
1st vaccination on 13 September 2021 with Janssen, batch number unknown, death 177 days later
2nd vaccination on 12 January 2022 with Comirnaty, batch number unknown, death 56 days later
Since the 2nd vaccination, the young man always felt a little ill and weak. He died on 9 March 2022.

Autopsy (forensic medicine)
No abnormalities on the corpse, no evidence of alcohol or drugs (toxicology). No previous illnesses, he was a smoker. SARS-CoV-2 smear was negative.

Cause of death: "Natural death from heart pump failure due to myocardial infarction." In the left descending coronary artery, a complete occlusion was found over 1.5 cm due to a soft blood clot. Pallor of the anterior wall of the heart as a feature of ischaemic heart damage that had already occurred some time ago. Subcutaneous fatty tissue of the thorax appears yellowish (diabetes?).

Acute myocardial infarction with recurrent myocardial infarctions. Severe changes in the entire vascular system, in particular the coronary arteries and the carotid artery and suspected diabetes. Fatty, soft vascular wall deposits in all coronary arteries and the vessels of the neck. Remarks: 24 year old young man, 66 kg, 175 cm.

Secondary pathohistological examination
There were clearly COVID-19 vaccine-associated organ changes, including a past and ongoing **myocarditis** with myocardial scars, but no atherosclerosis and no atheroma beds. In necrotic myocytes of scarred myocardial areas in particular, we were able to detect the **spike protein,** which is produced by body cells, through an immunohistochemical analysis. The nucleocapsid (even if weaker) and the beta-**amyloid** 1-42 protein were also immunohistochemically detectable in these cells. This protein was described in an experimental study as a binding partner of the S1 subunit of the spike protein and the ACE2 receptor, i.e. the receptor that is considered the docking receptor for the spike protein of the SARS-CoV-2 virus.
The detection of the nucleocapsid protein indicates an infection with the circulating wild virus, which may have occurred undetected before or after the COVID-19 vaccinations. The SARS-CoV-2 virus is normally harmless to young men and can therefore go unnoticed.
The immunohistochemical spike protein detection in necrotic areas of the heart muscle together with the signs of myocarditis that was already scarred in some areas of the heart at the time of death and still ongoing in others leads us to the conclusion that this severe myocarditis was essentially triggered by the COVID-19 vaccinations. In the brain, there was **microvasculitis of cerebral vessels** with residual haemorrhage. **Mediadissections** were found in the **aorta and a coronary artery** with cushion-shaped narrowing of the lumen due to hyaline swelling. This vascular damage is also repeatedly found in people who have died after COVID-19 vaccination.
The contribution of the preserved thrombus to the pathogenetic process is unclear due to the unknown sampling site. However, the autopsy report described a complete occlusion of more than 1.5 cm in the left descending coronary artery by a soft blood clot. Thrombus formation on the inflamed vessel wall of a coronary artery is imaginable here, which could have led to immediate death due to coronary artery occlusion (as in a heart attack).
The death is **almost certainly** a causal consequence of the COVID-19 vaccinations that have taken place.

C74

73y / m / 2x Com, 1x Mod, 1x Com / 311, 290, 101, 13

Death and vaccination history

1st vaccination on 17 March 2021 with Comirnaty EX8679, death 311 days later
2nd vaccination on 25 May 2021 with Comirnaty FD9234, death 290 days later
3rd vaccination on 10 December 2021 with Moderna Lot 000128A, death 101 days later
4th vaccination on 18 March 2022 with Comirnaty ACB9929, death 13 days later
Transfer from a gastroenterological to an internal intensive care unit for consultative insertion of a central venous catheter on 17 March 2022 (8 days before death). Vigilance reduction, partially soporous, comatose, laboured breathing with coarse crackling noices. Highly suspected herpes encephalitis treated with Acyclovir on cMRI. Empirical antibiotics.

Increasing respiratory insufficiency as time progressed, right-sided pneumonia on CT, protective intubation due to changing vigilance (GCS 7). Bronchoscopic examination showed a light-coloured, mucous secretion with evidence of MSSA short for Methicillin susceptible Staph. aureus. Severely stenosed aortic valve stenosis visible on TEE. In cCT cerebral oedema without signs of pressure. With further decompensation veno-venous ECMO, two hours later progressive pericardial effusion, hardly any improvement after puncture, circulatory collapse, resuscitation, death on 25 March 2022 at 6:13 pm.

Autopsy (pathology)

Cause of death: Left-sided global heart failure with extensive left ventricular acute myocardial infarction.

Pronounced generalised atherosclerosis with yellowish, hardened atheromatous beds in the endothelia. Pronounced coronary atherosclerosis with high-grade calcification of the branches of the anterior interventricular, circumflex and right coronary artery. RIVA and RCX with high-grade intimal sclerosis and significant to almost complete narrowing of the lumen. Condition following older infarcts in the area of the papillary muscle and older infarct scars elsewhere in the myocardium.

Minor generalised cerebral oedema in the substantia nigra of the brainstem and the basal ganglia.

Secondary pathohistological examination

The main underlying disease is generalised atherosclerosis with old and acute myocardial infarction foci. However, there were also **acute vasculitic changes** and protein material deposits in the myocardium and pancreas.

In the brain, pronounced inflammatory changes were found in the vessels of the brain substance and subarachnoid. The weak but clear **expression of spike protein in brain vessels** with a negative nucleocapsid speaks for a COVID-19 vaccine induced vasculitis in the arachnoid and brain tissue. As far as can be seen from the documents, herpes encephalitis was suspected and treated on the basis of MRI imaging, but not confirmed. In contrast, the changes found, suggest a high probability of vaccine/spike-induced vascular encephalitis.

In addition, textural disorders of the wall of the larger arteries, including the coronary arteries, with **elastic fibre fragmentation and elastic fibre destruction.** These COVID-19 vaccine associated vascular changes are likely to have been significantly involved in the death process in a severely pre-damaged vascular system.
In addition, there is a pronounced, florid **lymphocytic vasculitis and encephalitis,** which was spike protein toxic induced as indicated by the immunohistological spike protein detection. There was no reliable histopathological correlate for the clinically suspected herpes encephalitis; in particular, no nuclear inclusion bodies were found.
A connection of the death with the COVID-19 vaccination exists with a **probability bordering on certainty** due to the typical organ and vascular changes.

55y / m / 3x Com / 270, 210, 68 **C80**

Death and vaccination history

1st vaccination on 3 May 2021 with Comirnaty FA4598, death 270 days later
2nd vaccination on 2 July 2021 with Comirnaty FD6840, death 210 days later
3rd vaccination on 21 November 2021 with Comirnaty FJ5973, death 68 days later
Collapsed while walking. Layman and professional emergency resuscitation unsuccessful. The man died on 28 January 2022.

Autopsy (pathology)

Cause of death: Postvaccinal lymphocytic myocarditis. Pronounced interstitial myocardial oedema, dilatation of all cardiac cavities (heart weight 710 g), acute pulmonary congestion, pulmonary oedema, hypoxic brain damage after resuscitation, cholesteatosis of the gallbladder mucosa. Condition after 3 immunisations with Comirnaty. No significant coronary sclerotic changes. 1.80 cm tall, slightly obese body.

Secondary pathohistological examination

No significant signs of severe systemic pre-existing diseases such as atherosclerosis, but **pronounced COVID-19 vaccine-associated vascular changes** (microvasculitis in the brain, heart, skin and spleen). **Particle deposits** in the liver (here also intracellular), spleen, heart and pancreas. With regard to the (even if very weak) SARS-CoV-2 spike protein detection, the death is proven to be a consequence of the COVID-19 vaccination. The death is **almost certainly** a causal consequence of the 3 COVID-19 vaccinations that took place.

49y / f / 2x UNKN, 1x Com / xx, xx, 42 **C81**

History of death and vaccination

The woman received 3 COVID-19 vaccinations; however, the exact dates are not available in full.
1st vaccination: date unknown with UNKNOWN

2nd vaccination: date unknown with UNKNOWN
3rd vaccination/'booster' on 16 December 2021 with Comirnaty, death 42 days later
The 49-year-old died on 27 January 2022.

Autopsy (pathology)
Cause of death: Postvaccinal lymphocytic myocarditis, acute cerebral ventricular softening.

Secondary pathohistological examination
Histologically age-appropriate organs. No serious previous damage, in particular no severe atherosclerosis.
Apparently vaccine-induced microvasculitis with hyalinosis.
Deep **media necrosis and dissection of a coronary artery** with T-lymphocytic infiltration.
Lymphocyte-rich multifocal **myocarditis** with predominance of T-cells.
Multifocal deposits of black-brown, rod-shaped, non-localised material in the pancreas and spleen, but not in the heart and brain.
Death was **almost certainly** caused by COVID-19 vaccine-induced myocarditis and generalised vasculitis.

C82

40y / m / 1x UNKN / xx
History of death and vaccination
1st vaccination: Date unknown with UNKNOWN
The 40-year-old died on 28 January 2022. He was found lifeless in his flat.

Pathological report
Cause of death: instantaneous cardiac death due to lymphocytic myocarditis. 1.70 m tall, athletic, male corpse in normal nutritional condition.

Secondary pathohistological examination
Cause of death was probably a hyperacute myocardial infarction with subtotal coronary occlusion, which was obviously not atherosclerotic but caused by media-necrotic thickening of the inner vessel wall in the presence of **myocarditis.** SARS-CoV-2 immunohistochemistry was weakly positive in myocytes and endothelia, but we do not know which antigen was detected.
As we only had the microscope slides, but no specimens from which we could have prepared sections ourselves, we were unable to carry out any further immunohistochemical analyses.
However, the pathohisto-morphological picture of the **inflammatory vascular changes** in particular, corresponds to that which was repeatedly seen in people who died after COVID-19 vaccinations. The death was **almost certainly** caused by the COVID-19 vaccination.

C83

72y / m / 1x Astra, 1x Mod / 280, 196
History of death and vaccination
The 72-year-old died at home in the presence of his wife on the morning of 21 January 2022.
1st vaccination on 16 April 2021 with Astra Zeneca ABV5297, death 280 days later
2nd vaccination on 9 July 2021 with Moderna 3003603, death 196 days later
On 21 January 2022, the deceased asked his wife to take his blood pressure at around 10:15 am because he thought he was having a heart attack. Shortly afterwards, his head tilted back. Resuscitation was started immediately and the emergency physician arrived about 20 minutes later. Rapid breathing and ventricular fibrillation. Pre-hospital thrombolytics, intubation and mechanical ventilation. The man died under protracted resuscitation at 12:27 pm.
The relatives found a note in the trouser pocket of the deceased's clothing. According to the daughter-in-law, he had handwritten on it that he had had chest pains the previous evening and had taken an Aspirin tablet.
In November 2021, an ECG was performed at the family doctor's practice and the blood was analysed. When discussing the results of the autopsy, the family doctor again confirmed that all findings were without abnormalities.

Autopsy (pathology)
Cause of death: rhythmogenic heart failure.
Autopsy revealed biventricular, chronic ischaemic myocardial damage with severe general and coronary atherosclerosis as well as severe biventricular **myocardial hypertrophy** exceeding the critical heart weight (600 g), which in turn was caused by arterial hypertension with obesity (BMI 30 kg/m^2) and chronic nicotine abuse (cumulative 20 PY according to clinical data) with chronic obstructive pulmonary disease. A histo-morphological correlation of a clinically suspected myocardial infarction could not be confirmed by autopsy during preclinical thrombolytic therapy. Early microscopic changes of a myocardial infarction appear after approx. 6 hours. It is possible that this time interval was not reached in the present case, so that microscopically detectable changes of a myocardial infarction were not yet present.

Secondary pathohistological examination
The histological findings of the initial pathological examination were basically confirmed. The main changes were also confirmed in the coronary arteries (pronounced arteriosclerosis) and the heart muscle (heart weight 600 g) with discordant hypertrophy and individual scars. There is therefore no doubt that the heart is severely damaged.
In addition, however, isolated interstitial lymphocytes and a discrete lymphocytic epicarditis were detected. This finding is suggestive of a vaccination episode.
In the available **coronary artery** sections, considerable arteriosclerosis and atheromatosis were confirmed. In addition, however, perivascular circumscribed haemorrhages, **deep media necrosis with dissection** and discrete vasculitis of the vasa vasorum were found. These changes, which cannot otherwise be found in banal coronary

sclerosis, are also seen in terms of vaccination/spike protein induced vascular damage. Only fragments of **elastic fibres** are preserved, no continuous fibre structure is visible. In the area of the medial dissection, the spike protein can be detected immunohistochemically in inflammatory cells, especially in mononuclear phagocytes.
The **granular and rod-shaped, brownish, non-localised particles** in the heart and liver were not described by the previous investigators. These are also frequently detected in people who have died in connection with COVID-19 vaccination. Their significance and their influence on the death process are still unclear. The spleen was not examined histologically, although typical manifestations of spike protein induced tissue damage can be found in the spleen. The brain was only assessed macroscopically and no histological examination with assessment of the large and small cerebral vessels was performed. Accordingly, we did not have any histological samples from the brain.
In view of the massive damage to the coronary artery that typically occurs after COVID-19 vaccinations (media necrosis with destruction of the elastic fibres and detection of the spike protein), there is **almost certainly** a connection between the COVID-19 vaccinations that took place and the death.

C85

22y / m / 1x Jan, 1x Com / 364, 238
History of death and vaccination
The 22-year-old shot himself on 25 August 2022 as a result of a myocarditis diagnosis with corresponding loss of performance and quality of life.
1st vaccination on 26 August 2021 with Janssen 21C18-03, death 364 days later
2nd vaccination on 30 December 2021 with Comirnaty PCA0003, death 238 days later
After the vaccinations, the young man experienced a sharp drop in performance in everyday life and also as a competitive swimmer. The medical diagnosis of myocarditis with the prognosis of permanently severely reduced performance prompted him to buy a gun, which was registered on 22 August 2022. 3 days later, on 25 August 2022, he killed himself by shooting himself in the mouth.

Autopsy (pathology)
Cause of death: suicide by pistol shot.
The second opinion was delivered by Burkhardt and Lang to pathohistologically verify the clinically diagnosed myocarditis that motivated the suicide.

Secondary pathohistological examination
The main finding in the deceased was **severe,** partly florid, partly subsided and scarring **myocarditis** with an existing acute episode at the time of death. The scarring was centred in the right ventricle.
There was a multifocal event in the myocardium. An infarction can be ruled out as the cause of the scarring:

- no coronary sclerosis
- multifocality
- predominantly lymphocytic infiltrates.

Clear textural distorsions of the walls of large arteries and the aorta with media swelling and discrete inflammation of the vasa vasorum. Discrete perivasculitis in the skin and an (only slightly pronounced) 'onion skin phenomenon' of the splenic arteries fit into the picture.
It is **almost certain** that severe COVID-19 vaccine-related organ damage was present at the time of the suicide. This is confirmed by the **positive spike protein** detection in the damaged organ structures, especially myocardium, coronary arteries and aorta, with negative findings for nucleocapsid immunohistochemistry.

74y / m / 3x Com / 400, 367, 156 **C91**

History of death and vaccination

The 74-year-old died on 15 October 2022 in the hospital where he had been hospitalised due to previous, recurrent motor weakness and deficits. He suffered occasional falls.
1st vaccination on 10 September 2021 with Comirnaty SCKT8, death 400 days later
2nd vaccination on 13 October 2021 with Comirnaty 1H049A, death 367 days later
3rd vaccination on 12 May 2022 with Comirnaty 34396TB, death 156 days later
On the day of death, after going to the toilet, which he managed without any problems with the help of a nurse or his partner, the 74-year-old suddenly turned "bright red in the face and then completely white". The nurse responded with administration of oxygen before the doctor arrived. He then had another similar episode at around 4 pm, but it ended just as quickly as the previous one.
At around 7 pm, another syncope occurred, this time with a rapid drop in blood pressure to RR 80/40. Shortly afterwards, his partner could no longer feel his pulse. The 45-minute resuscitation was unsuccessful.

Medical history

Overweight with well-controlled high blood pressure. He had a minor stroke in February 2019, which was "resolved so far" after a 2-day hospital stay in South Africa. He was left with a slight discomfort in his left arm, but no other complaints.

Autopsy (pathology)

Cause of death: Fulminant bilateral **pulmonary artery embolism** and acute cor pulmonale with fresh thrombi in the right lower and femoral veins.
Autopsy findings: Severe cardiac hypertrophy (665 g), in particular with hypertrophy of the left ventricle and dilatation of both ventricles, emphasising the right ventricle (cor pulmonale). Pronounced coronary sclerosis, but no evidence of a recent or older myocardial infarction. Reticular callus formation sub-endocardially in the area of the left posterior wall. Degenerative changes to the mitral valve. Severe arteriosclerosis, particularly in the area of the abdominal aorta and in the area of the left external carotid artery with open plaque formation.
Fresh thrombus in the area of the right lower leg veins and the right femoral vein. Left lower leg was fine.

Fulminant pulmonary embolisms on both sides with obstruction of all large pulmonary arteries. No pulmonary infarctions.

Secondary pathohistological examination
In addition to pronounced, partially calcifying atherosclerosis, there were **textural disorders of the large and small vessels,** as observed after COVID-19 vaccinations. Necrotising myositis in the right lower leg with fresh thrombus formation in the adjacent veins. An embolus was obviously carried from this area into the lungs. The thrombus may have formed as part of the myositis.
Due to the positive spike protein detection in several vessels, including a coronary artery with medial dissection, it can be assumed with a **probability bordering on certainty** that vaccine/spike protein induced myositis with thrombosis was the starting point of a fatal pulmonary artery embolism.

C103

47y / m / UNKN / xx
History of death and vaccination
Relatives suspect that vaccinations were given during his hospitalisation. No documentation regarding COVID-19 vaccinations.

Medical history
Known psychosis since adolescence, suicide attempt in 2015 with numerous self-inflicted knife wounds with corresponding permanent damage.

- Stabbed abdominal organs with adhesions since 2015
- Pulmonary artery embolism 2015

On 17 June 2022 median laparotomy for abdominal wall reconstruction with mesh insertion. Large plastic mesh (30 x 20 cm) spread between the layers of the abdominal muscles. Death 10 days later, on 27 June 2022.

Post-mortem examination (forensic medicine)
47-year-old male, 118 kg, 182 cm.
Cause of death: Fulminant pulmonary embolism due to postoperative leg vein thrombosis.

- Various adhesions and adhesions of the intestinal loops to each other. Condition after appendectomy. Postoperative paralytic ileus.
- No acute relevant signs of inflammation, no abscesses anywhere. Regular wound conditions.
- Condition after intensive care immobilisation.
- Very extensive leg vein thromboses on both sides (femoral vein with secondary branches, extensive calf vein thromboses).
- Pronounced, acute, fulminant pulmonary embolisms: bulging, typical clots (probably from the femoral veins) in the arteries of the lung lobes. Smaller peripheral pulmonary emboli. No demarcated pulmonary infarction.

- Signs of acute myocardial failure with prominent right heart failure.
- Apart from the thromboses and the washed-in clots, liquid corpse blood, pronounced generalised cyanosis.
- Considerable fatty liver.
- Chronic arterial hypertension. Generalised heart enlargement, heart weight 590 g.
- Minor general arteriosclerosis (lipoidosis), minor coronary arteriosclerosis, no relevant stenosis, no thrombosis.

Secondary pathohistological examination
The **positive spike protein detection** in the large femoral vessels and the **particle deposits in the pancreas** indicate that COVID-19 vaccinations have taken place. The **thrombosis** in the femoral vein was probably due to spike protein induced endothelial damage. We have no histological specimen of the apparently directly fatal pulmonary embolism.
It is therefore **likely** that a COVID-19 vaccination was involved in the development of the disease.

C104

73y / f / 2x Com, 1x Mod / 366, 324, 103
History of death and vaccination
1st vaccination on 10 April 2021 with Comirnaty EW8904, death 366 days later
2nd vaccination on 22 May 2021 with Comirnaty 1C008A, death 324 days later
3rd vaccination on 29 December 2021 with Moderna 000110A, death 103 days later
The 73-year-old woman was found sitting dead on the couch by her son on 11 April 2022. Due to the rigor mortis that had already set in, no resuscitation attempts were made.

Son's report on the state of health of the deceased
"Unfortunately, I do not have any relevant medical reports. However, I do know that my mother had diabetes and blood pressure problems, which was actually well controlled with medication. She took part in social life as normal, attended the senior citizens' club, a dance and painting class, helped my brother's family by looking after their children or driving them to afternoon events every week. As I live further away with my family, we didn't see each other that often, maybe every two to six months, but she always seemed as fit as ever. Two days before she died, I spoke to her on the phone to tell her that we were going on holiday relatively spontaneously. We had a cheerful, relaxed conversation and she didn't seem to have any health problems.
From our point of view, she could easily have lived for another 10 years because she actually seemed fit. Her death therefore seemed surprising and completely unforeseeable to us, which is why we requested a forensic post-mortem examination."

Forensic examination
73-year-old woman, 74 kg, 162 cm.

Cause of death: Acute pumping failure of the heart with pericardial blood tamponade as a result of a ruptured myocardial infarction caused by an occlusion of the anterior descending branch of the left coronary artery (2 cm long, complete obliterative occlusion).

Secondary pathohistological examination
Atherosclerosis of varying severity. Known diabetes. Aorta and large vessels with mild, but marked atherosclerosis in the myocardial vessels and basal cerebral arteries. Stenosing coronary artery sclerosis, but additional deep and especially in the arterioles of the myocardium **endothelialitis** and stenosing hyaline vessel wall deposits, questionable amyloid or fibrinoid amyloid.
Only discrete myocardial callosities, no extensive older infarcts. No acute myocardial necrosis was detectable in the analysed specimens. Discrete epicarditis. There are two competing vascular changes: On the one hand, severe vascular stenosing atherosclerosis, on the other hand, a probable spike protein induced textural disorder on the vessel walls of the aorta and myocardial vessels. Stenosing endothelialitis with hyaline wall deposits of the myocardium.
A summation of the atherosclerotic-induced reduced supply of the myocardium and spike protein related vascular changes with disruption of the microcirculation may be the cause of the myocardial wall rupture, which we were unable to verify.
The **amyloid deposits** in the arterioles of the spleen and myocardium were confirmed by Congo red staining. Spike protein presence in the fibrinoid/amyloid material could indicate fibrin-amyloid spike protein complexes. No signs of spike protein in the aorta. The last COVID-19 vaccination was 103 days ago, which could already have caused the degradation here.
In addition, there is multifocal chronic interstitial pneumonia, often with tissue destruction and formation of cholesterol crystals with attached giant cells. Dense, round cell infiltrations in the interstitial spaces and massive alveolar macrophage proliferation.
Deposits of non-localised material were found in the liver.
A connection with the COVID-19 vaccinations that took place is **probable.**

C108

59y / f / no vaccinations, suspected shedding transmission by relatives
History of death and vaccination
No COVID-19 vaccinations received. Relatives express suspicion of shedding.
The 59-year-old woman was found dead in bed on 19 September 2022 in the morning. The family suspects an indirect COVID-19 vaccination episode consistent with shedding or a Long COVID episode (COVID-19 infection in March/April 2022, 6 months before death).
The 59-year-old had been increasingly unwell for several months. She had been suffering from back pain, among other things. The family saw parallels to the clinical picture of what is commonly referred to as Long COVID.

A son had been diagnosed with a COVID-19 infection five months earlier. As a result, the 59-year-old was also "flu-like" and subsequently became increasingly tired, fatigued and had back pain. Many household contacts with COVID-19 vaccinated people, e.g. in the household where the woman worked.

Autopsy report (forensic medicine)
Woman, 59 years old, 168 cm, 83 kg.
Cause of death: Basically compatible with sudden cardiac death with severe thickening of the heart muscle.
There was clearly pre-damage to the heart in the form of an increase in muscular mass and thickening. This may be the result of untreated high blood pressure or an independent disease (hypertrophic cardiomyopathy). The whitish thickening of the inner lining of the left heart was also conspicuous. This could also be an independent clinical picture. These findings of the heart alone can explain a deterioration in health over a longer period of time. The chequered pattern on the heart muscle section may be the result of the resuscitation that took place on the basis of the findings.
Histological examinations can clarify whether myocarditis is present.
The pre-existing heart disease should not be regarded as the result of immunisation or shedding. Most likely natural death.

Secondary pathohistological examination
Endocardial fibrosis, minimal endocarditis, minimal lymphocytic epicarditis. Hyaline swelling of vessels. Dissection and minimal **endothelialitis** of the coronary arteries. **Spike protein markings** in the vessel wall (endothelium, myofibroblasts and surrounding inflammatory cells) with negative nucleocapsid.
Uncertain particles in the pancreas, myocardium and at one site in the lungs.
The discrete epicarditis and the sometimes more pronounced textural distorsions of the vessels would be compatible with spike protein/COVID-19 vaccine-associated lesions, but may also be associated with a natural infection. **Relationships unclear.**

40y / m / UNKN / xx **C111**
History of death and vaccination
An unsuccessful attempt was made to read the app on the decommissioned mobile phone. **The vaccination card itself had been thrown away.**
Died in the swimming pool on 15 February 2022. The 40-year-old was in the swimming pool to train for a triathlon. After 100 metres, he told his training partner that he had a calf cramp. He then supported himself briefly on the edge of the pool with his arms and slipped unconscious into the water. Resuscitation attempts were unsuccessful.

Post-mortem examination (forensic medicine)
40-year-old man, 187 cm, 74 kg.

The post-mortem report is not very informative. The autopsy report was requested from the father. It is also possible that there is no further report. Perhaps not much could be recognised macroscopically.
Heart weight 560 g, this was described by forensic medicine as exceeding the critical heart mass, but the deceased was above average height at 187 cm and apparently also athletic.

Secondary pathohistological examination
Not quite acute, already scarred, diffuse, focal **myocarditis** with multiple, acute muscle fibre infiltrations with surrounding leukocytic infiltration, mainly lymphocytes and macrophages. **Endothelialitis** of arterioles. Vacuolar focal deposits of particles not further defined. The findings would be compatible with a COVID-19 vaccine related myocarditis, whereby the first vaccination would have to be at least 8 weeks ago. Minimal lymphocytic vasculitis in the brain. Sections of coronary arteries without atherosclerosis, but with age-typical fibromuscular beds and lymphocytic perivasculitis. Furthermore, positive **spike protein detection** predominantly in endothelia of the myocardial vessels and pronounced spike protein-associated elasticity destruction. Detected in the heart, coronary arteries and small cerebral vessels. Partly healed, partly florid myocarditis must be considered the cause of death.
A connection with the COVID-19 vaccinations is **almost certain.** This is supported by the spike markings in the myocardium, especially in the arteriolar walls, as well as by the pronounced **elastic destruction** in the vascular walls of the heart and brain. Furthermore, particle deposits were found in the heart.

C128

29y / f / 1x Com / 21
History of death and vaccination
1st vaccination on 4 April 2021 with Comirnaty, batch number unknown, death 21 days later
Collapsed in the morning with cardiovascular arrest. Massive aspiration during on-site resuscitation. After suctioning, intubation, Fenistil, Prednisolone and Suprarenin, emergency admission with continuation of resuscitation measures (bag ventilation).
Emergency laboratory abnormalities:

- Hb 7.0; platelets 27x103/µL (Ref 220-406); leukocytes 2.5 x 103/µL (Ref 4.4-11.3), thus signs of anaemia, thrombocytopenia and leukocytopenia
- Quick (coagulation) 11 %; norm 70 – 100 %
- Hypoalbuminaemia 1.4 g/dL; norm 3.4-4.8 g/dL

A haematopoietic disorder was not previously known.
Death in the intensive care unit on 25 April 2021 after unsuccessful medical catecholamine-resistant resuscitation.

Medical history

- Multiple sclerosis (stable with 14-day Plegridy antibody treatment)
- Asthma
- Severe cross allergy to nuts and apples

An investigation was initiated.

Post-mortem examination (forensic medicine)

Body of a 29-year-old woman, 164 cm, 59 kg.
Heart: signs of chronic lymphocytic myocarditis with oedema and focally accentuated areas of fibrosis.
Bone marrow regularly haematopoietic.
Pharyngeal mucosa oedematous with inflammatory infiltration by eosinophilic granulocytes and occasional mast cells. This can be interpreted as correlating to an allergic reaction.
The forensic expert's report does not comment on a possible connection with the COVID-19 vaccination that had taken place 21 days before death. The following wording can be found in the letter from the public prosecutor's office on the preliminary proceedings referring to this report: "A causality of the COVID-19 vaccination for the onset of death could not be established."

Secondary pathohistological examination

The myocarditis already diagnosed by forensic medicine is confirmed. The **myocarditis** is accompanied by clear **positivity of spike protein** in the intramural blood vessels of the heart and in myocardial fibres – negative nucleocapsid immunohistochemistry. Thus, the COVID-19 vaccination that had taken place 21 days earlier can be seen as the cause of the myocarditis.
Spike proteins were also detected in the pharyngeal tonsils. However, the inflammatory process in the pharyngeal tonsils is not related to the death.
The whole brain in formalin was sent to us and handed over to a neuropathology department. This essentially concerns the neuropathological confirmation of the pre-existing multiple sclerosis. However, we do not expect any additional information regarding the cause of death due to the COVID-19 vaccination.
The COVID-19 vaccination **almost certainly** led to cardiac death.

60y / m / 1x Jan / 61 **C138**

History of death and vaccination

1st vaccination on 20 September 2021 with Janssen 21C16-01, death 61 days later
According to the brother, who also arranged the autopsy, the 60-year-old man experienced an immediate drop in performance after the COVID-19 vaccination, which was accompanied by weight gain; he had no known previous illnesses and had been very active as a hiking guide.
Collapsed on 5 November 2021 and died after unsuccessful resuscitation. Suspected Th4 syndrome (back and cervical spine pain syndrome).

Post-mortem examination (pathology)
Male corpse, 169 cm, 80 kg.
Medical history: condition after pleurisy, also paraesthesia in the right arm since 2016. About 4 years ago suspected lower leg thrombosis without medical treatment. Recent circulatory disorders of the extremities. In recent months, shortness of breath at night, nosebleeds.
Acute shortness of breath two days before death. Outpatient medical examination revealed high blood pressure, inpatient treatment refused.
Cause of death: Fulminant bilateral pulmonary embolism in recurrent leg vein thrombosis with right ventricular circulatory failure.
The immediate cause of death was thrombi with older and fresh parts in the central pulmonary arteries on both sides. In addition, there was evidence of expired deep vein thrombosis in the legs, which therefore represent the probable starting point of the pulmonary embolisms.
Further **main findings:**

- Left ventricular cardiac hypertrophy with age-related mild atherosclerosis
- Minor intra-alveolar siderosis
- Initial benign glomerulosclerosis as a feature of chronic arterial hypertension

Secondary findings: fatty liver (30 %), initial, subpleural emphysema, small goitre colloides nodosa.
"A connection with the COVID vaccination given approx. 9 weeks previously and therefore some time ago seems unlikely."

Secondary pathohistological examination
A not quite fresh **thrombus** and perivascular abscessing inflammation were found in a larger pulmonary artery. No pulmonary infarction in the samples examined, but disseminated granuloma formations and lymphocytic perivasculitis in the lungs. Partly compact, partly rod-shaped **particle deposits** with birefringence in various organs (heart, lung, kidney, adrenal gland, pancreas, gastrointestinal mucosa).
Focal active chronic **myocarditis** with mild activity. Pronounced particle deposits, as frequently observed after COVID-19 vaccinations. Histomorphological evidence of the vaccination.
A significant contribution of the COVID-19 vaccination to the death is **probable,** but cannot be proven.

C139

59y / m / 3x Com / 417, 380, 242
History of death and vaccination
1st vaccination on 3 June 2021 with Comirnaty 1C011A, death 417 days later
2nd vaccination on 10 July 2021 with Comirnaty FC1440, death 380 days later
3rd vaccination on 25 November 2021 with Comirnaty SDEWS, death 242 days later
The deceased had been complaining about back pain since February 2022. On 18 July he went to hospital due to his poor condition. There he was found to have:

- Thrombosis and inflammation of the heart valves. A CT scan showed an enlarged spleen and thrombi in the liver and kidneys.
- On 23 July, loss of consciousness, cerebral haemorrhage detectable on CT, transfer to the neurology department, emergency surgery was performed to relieve pressure.

Death on 25 July 2022 (ventilation was switched off due to the destruction of large areas of the brain).

Autopsy (pathology and neuropathology)
Clinical data: Endocarditis > cerebral ischaemia > haemorrhage > evacuation ICB > secondary haemorrhage (SDH + EPH) > intracranial pressure > incarceration > brain death
Cause of death: death due to right-sided ventricular haemorrhage with intracranial haemorrhages.
Further pathological anatomical diagnoses:

- Endocarditis of the mitral valve due to degenerative changes
- Septic embolisms in the subclavian artery and in the left lower lobe of the lung
- Haemorrhages and partial areas of infarction in the brain can be the residue of septic emboli without detectable pathogens. However, there are no typical patterns of spread of septic emboli or septic infarcts into the brain.
- Thrombosis of the lower leg on both sides
- Splenic infarction
- Pleural effusion
- Pericardial effusion
- Shock kidneys
- Pulmonary haemorrhage, oedema, emphysema

Secondary diagnoses: Hyperplastic thyroid nodules on both sides, sigmoid diverticulum, haemangioma of the spine.
Comment: To rule out congophilic angiopathy with certainty, the material would have to be examined by reference pathology. This may incur additional costs. If this is desired, please let us know. There are no specific indications of a connection with vaccination against COVID-19 over 6 months ago.

Secondary pathohistological examination
There are several organ lesions, which in themselves could be a possible cause of death.
Ultimately, an acute multilocular **cerebral** haemorrhage **and** a **subarachnoid haemorrhage** probably led to death. This was most probably due to a spike protein toxic microangiopathy with destruction of elastic layers. An apparently fresh haemorrhage without haemosiderin deposition was found in the brain.
In addition, however, there was a severe **myocarditis** with endocarditis that had progressed over several years, which in itself would be a sufficient cause of death. There is no evidence of a bacterial toxic event. In addition, a not quite acute splenic infarction with perisplenitis and a small fresh embolus in the lung was found.

The death was **almost certainly** caused by the well-documented vascular damage typical of COVID-19 vaccination and myocarditis. This is further confirmed by the positive spike protein detection and the inflammatory infiltrates of the myocarditis.

C152

21y / m / 2x Com / 170, 130
History of death and vaccination
1st vaccination on 10 April 2021 with Comirnaty FC3095, death 170 days later
2nd vaccination on 20 May 2021 with Comirnaty FE6975, death 130 days later
On the day of death, 27 September 2021, the 21-year-old went out with 2 friends but did not return. Instead, he was found lying on his back later that afternoon. Resuscitation, which was started immediately and continued by the emergency services, was unsuccessful.
According to the family, the deceased had already been unwell on the morning of the day of his death, complaining of chest pains and loss of appetite. No previous illnesses, no medication (apart from the COVID-19 vaccinations).

Post-mortem examination (forensic medicine)
21-year-old man, 183 cm, 109 kg.
Increased heart weight (520 g). Left and right heart hypertrophy, suspected acute myocardial hypertrophy. Lidocaine was found in high concentrations in forensic medicine (probably administered by the emergency physician). Spleen 450 g, liver 2770 g.

Secondary pathohistological examination
There were no histopathological findings in the organs that could explain the sudden death. No spike protein could be detected in the myocardium. Deposits of small, crystalline rod-shaped, intravacuolar particles were found in some myocardial sections and in sections of the pancreas.
A connection between the sudden death and the COVID-19 vaccinations can **neither be proven nor ruled out.**

C159

16y / f / 2x Com / 58, 26
History of death and vaccination
1st vaccination on 8 June 2021 presumably with Comirnaty, batch number unknown, death 58 days later
2nd vaccination on 10 July 2021 with Comirnaty, batch number unknown, death 26 days later
14 days after the 1st vaccination presentation at the vaccinator's GP surgery due to general weakness and back pain. Treatment with Buscopan and Ibuprophen.
Three days after the 2nd vaccination, the patient reported pain in her right arm. On 15 July (5 days after the vaccination), the patient collapsed. After one hour of

resuscitation and emergency medical care, intensive medical care was provided in hospital.
In the further course, oxygen deficiency damage to the brain, renal insufficiency and deep thrombosis of the left-sided arm veins with swelling of the left arm were diagnosed.
On 23 July 2021, tissue samples were taken from the right ventricle during a cardiac catheterisation. The histological examination of the biopsies revealed a "moderate degree of chronic myocardial damage with interstitial remodelling of the myocardium and an increased deposition of macrophages", whereby the chronic damage to the heart muscle could have been the result of a long-standing inflammatory reaction or a congenital, genetically determined damage to the metabolism of the muscle cells.
The condition of the person concerned had deteriorated; she finally died on 5 August 2021 as a result of "hyperkalaemia" following "hypoxic kidney damage".
No previous illnesses were known, but the patient had recently been increasingly listless and tired.

Autopsy

- Older, haemorrhaged myocardial necrosis in the ventricular septum and in the muscles of the bicuspid leaflet valve.
- Older accumulation of blood in the pericardium (approx. 270 ml) after biopsy of the right ventricle on 23 July 2021, known from previous history.
- Signs of severe oxygen deficiency damage to the brain tissue with cerebral oedema and signs of intracranial pressure.
- Inflammatory changes in the respiratory organs.
- Pulmonary oedema.
- Septic softening of the enlarged spleen (organ weight 362 g).
- Flaccid consistency of the enlarged liver and cloudy swelling of the kidneys.
- Signs of **generalised blood coagulation disorder.**
- Abdominal and thoracic cavity effusions on both sides.
- **Thrombotic occlusion** of the left subclavian and brachial veins.
- Generalised, low-grade arteriosclerosis.

Fine tissue examination:

- Pronounced interstitial pneumonia with bacterial superinfection (bronchopneumonia).
- Severe chronic damage to the myocardium as in active chronic myocarditis with partial extensive necrosis of the myocardium consistent with an acute exacerbation.
- Cerebral oedema and disseminated ganglion and Purkinje cell necrosis.
- Generalised congestion of the internal organs.
- Fresh, non-historical thrombus (less than two weeks old) of the subclavian vein.

Preliminary autopsy report from the forensic medicine department

The histological and immunohistological findings show a moderate degree of chronic myocardial damage with interstitial remodeling of the myocardium and an increased deposition of macrophages.
The **cause of death** was stated in the 'preliminary autopsy report' as septic-toxic multi-organ failure with inflammatory changes in the respiratory organs. The organ failure in turn was considered to be an indirect consequence of the hypoxic brain damage, which could be explained by the cardiovascular arrest on 15 July 2021 known from the previous history.

Secondary pathohistological examination

In the foreground were the findings on the myocardium with partly weeks-old, partly days-old foci of necrosis, consistent with a chronic **myocarditis.** In myocardial fibres and in capillary endothelia of the myocardium, **spike protein markings** were clearly visible with negative nucleocapsid.
Multiple abscessing inflammatory foci were detectable in the lungs, which must also have been involved in the death process.
In view of the autopsy findings, the detection of the vaccine-induced spike protein and the symptoms described by the deceased after the two vaccinations, and in line with the current scientific literature available, the two vaccinations with Corminaty are **almost certainly** the cause of death, especially as there were no relevant pre-existing conditions in the adolescent.

C160

54y / m / 2x Com, 1x Mod, 1x Com / 641, 622, 426, 144

History of death and vaccination

1st vaccination on 14 May 2021 with Comirnaty EX8679, death 641 days later
2nd vaccination on 2 June 2021 with Comirnaty FC3095, death 622 days later
3rd vaccination on 15 December 2021 with Moderna Lot 3004233, death 426 days later
4th vaccination on 23 September 2022 with Comirnaty GH9715, death 144 days later

Medical history

- Systemic lupus erythematosus (SLE)
- Polyarthritis
- Arterial hypertension
- Coronary heart disease
- Hashimoto's thyroiditis
- Atrial fibrillation with intake of Eliquis (Apixaban thrombokinase inhibitor)
- Condition after total hip replacement.

From one week after the 4th COVID-19 vaccination (on 23 September 2022) almost continuously ill, especially dyspnoea on exertion.
At the end of October 2022, a peripheral pulmonary embolism was diagnosed on both sides by CT, which led to a 4-week hospitalisation. These pulmonary embolisms

occurred while taking anticoagulants due to atrial fibrillation for approx. 6 months. The medication was switched to Marcumar in hospital. This was followed by an unexplained fever in the afternoon. No tumour or infection could be found.
A relapse of SLE was suspected and treated with cortisone. In the meantime, a urinary tract infection was diagnosed and treated with antibiotics.
In January 2023, persistent shortness of breath with pleural effusions; diuretics and pleural puncture treatment.
Chest CT morphologically like "Covid lung", but COVID-19 PCR and rapid test negative.
Bronchoscopy for pathogen diagnosis initially inconclusive.
High-dose cortisone (due to SLE) brings little improvement.
Impending kidney failure → dialysis treatment.
On 2 February 2023 (11 days before death) tonic-clonic seizure, evidence of temporal lobe haemorrhage. In the neurological intensive care unit, high doses of catecholamines with severe side effects (necrosis of the fingertips), erythrocyte concentrates and nosocomial pathogens in the bronchial secretions (P. aeruginosa, K. pneumoniae).
Fulminant course with septic shock and multi-organ failure under triple antibiotics.
Death on 13 February 2023.

Autopsy (pathology)
Cause of death: Multi-organ failure in the context of diffuse alveolar haemorrhage, exacerbated by a severely chronic, pre-damaged lung with cerebral haemorrhagic infarction with ischaemia.
Main diagnoses
Diffuse alveolar haemorrhage with signs of protracted shock
- Desquamation of the alveolar surface cell layer with haemorrhagic lung parenchyma
- Shock kidneys with cortical marrow demarcation
- Haemostasis of parenchymal organs
- Disintegrating splenic parenchyma
- Serous ascites (200 ml), icterus
- **Multiple cerebral haemorrhages with haemorrhagic infarctions** and 6 x 4 x 3.5 cm parenchymal defect in the temporal lobe consistent with a haemorrhagic infarction (neuropathological report)

Pulmonary accentuated signs of SLE
- Pleuritis with thickened pleural sheets
- Severe interstitial lung disease with massive fibrotic aspect, metaplastic bone neoplasms and formation of hyaline membranes in the lung parenchyma as well as chronic lympho-plasmacytic inflammatory reaction
- Mild glomerulosclerosis

Signs of chronic damage to the heart
- Left ventricular myocardial hypertrophy (heart weight 550 g, myocardial thickness left 1.9 cm)
- Interstitial fibrosis and chronic infarct areas
- Moderate-grade coronary sclerosis with lumen obliteration of 20 %

Moderate to high-grade atherosclerosis with infrarenal emphasis
- Plaques of the aorta with infrarenal emphasis

Secondary diagnoses: Meckel's diverticulum, mild thyroiditis, cholecystolithiasis and choledocholithiasis

Secondary pathohistological examination
In addition to scarring in the myocardium, an acute round-cell infiltration was occasionally detectable, suggesting the possibility of **lymphocytic myocarditis.** The immunohistochemical examination for the **spike protein** revealed a clear **positivity** in the capillary endothelia of the myocardial interstitium as well as in the endothelia of the vessels of the subepicardial fatty tissue.
The suspected diagnosis of interstitial pulmonary fibrosis made by the pathologist was mild and not indicative of systemic lung disease based on our histochemical examinations. Immunohistochemical testing for the spike protein showed clear positivity in the alveolar macrophages and type II pneumocytes and weak positivity in the vascular endothelia.
Hashimoto's thyroiditis can be ruled out in the present study. Our investigations are in favour of postvaccinal lesions in the myocardium and lungs.
Thus, there is a **high probability** that the death was related to the COVID-19 vaccinations that took place.

C164

72y / f / 6x UNKN / xx, xx, xx, xx, xx, xx
Death and vaccination history
"Vaccinated 3x, boostered 3x." 72 year old woman found dead in bed on 2 April 2023. Private autopsy was performed. Some time before death, the woman complained of fatigue and coughing.

Post-mortem examination (forensic medicine)
Main diagnoses
- Cardiomegaly (600 g) with short stature
- End-stage dilated cardiomyopathy, dysfunctional AV valves
- Generalised coronary stenosis, "occluded vessels" – accumulation of fluid in the pericardium and chest cavity was considered a feature of a longstanding disease process (decompensatio cordis)

Conclusion: Acute fatal infarction in a severely pre-damaged heart.
Histology: Significant fibrosis and hypertrophy features. No signs of ‚dysarray'. Contraction band necrosis and eosinophilic degeneration are mainly observed in the papillary muscle fields with dissolved contractile tissue. Fields with hypertrophy nuclei. Significant granulocyte and lymphocyte proliferation between the myocardial fibres, especially in the vessels. The increase in lipofuscin pigment is striking.
Conclusion: Highly preloaded myocardium with signs of persistent hypoxia and recent ischaemia. Possible signs of lymphatic activity.

Secondary pathohistological examination

The specimens were 3 myocardial sections. A comprehensive pathohistological assessment was not possible due to the sparse information and the small number of specimens.
Myocardium 1: No necrosis. No signs of interstitial inflammation.
Myocardium 2: Small focal fibrosis and minor round cell infiltration. No spike protein markings detectable.
Myocardium 3: Small-centre scarring. No interstitial inflammation, no necrosis.
No spike protein markings could be detected by immunohistochemistry. Due to the inadequate sampling of the myocardium by forensic medicine, a diagnosis of vaccine-induced myocarditis due to spike toxicity was not possible. Furthermore, a follow-up examination was impossible because the organs were not preserved.

61y / m / 2x Com / 123, 98 **Ext**

History of death and vaccination

61-year-old multi morbid man died after a one-month stay in hospital on 8 October 2021. A clinical autopsy was arranged.
1st vaccination on 7 June 2021 with Comirnaty EW5279, death 123 days later
2nd vaccination on 2 July 2021 with Comirnaty FA8016, death 98 days later
The patient received two doses of the vaccine between two treatment periods of cytostatic therapy combined with Rituximab.

Medical history

Several malignancies had been diagnosed in the six years prior to death. Among others, a thyroid carcinoma was diagnosed, which was treated with a total thyroidectomy. A prostate carcinoma was treated with prostatectomy. A recurrent follicular B-cell lymphoma had to be treated repeatedly with chemotherapy, the last four chemotherapies in combination with Rituximab. The patient initially recovered from the last recurrence of the lymphoma and the imaging procedures showed a reduction in the tumour volume. However, a few days after the last chemotherapy and two months after the second vaccination, the patient was hospitalised with an acute infection. Soon afterwards, he developed liver failure and a picture of Guillain-Barré syndrome (GBS) with acute polyneuropathy with weakness in the arms and legs as well as bilateral facial nerve palsy.

Autopsy (pathology)

Cause of death: Signs of acute liver failure and vasculitis with acute cerebral infarction in the medulla oblongata.
Main findings: Massive myeloradiculitis and T-cell infiltrates in the brain, liver, pancreas and kidneys.

Pathohistological examination

The liver showed confluent, centrilobular necrosis and a pronounced, lobular centrally accentuated intra- and extracellular cholestasis. The kidneys showed the picture of a cholestatic nephropathy.

In the brain, lymphoid perivascular cell infiltrates were found in the frontal and temporal lobes and the medulla oblongata. In the corpus callosum and the medulla oblongata, a focal picture of vasculitis with surrounding acute cerebral infarcts of up to 4 mm in diameter was seen.

Based on the clinically described GBS, the spinal cord, the neighbouring radicular nerves and the axillary nerves were examined. Histopathologically, a dense lymphatic infiltrate was found in the radicular nerves intra- and perineurally with decreasing intensity from cervical to lumbar.

In the spinal cord there were isolated lymphoid infiltrates, especially perivascular. A loose lymphoid cell infiltrate was seen in the axillary nerve sections, which was also partially detectable perineurally.

Patchy lymphocytic infiltrates were also found in the liver, kidneys and pancreas. Immunohistochemically, the lymphocytic infiltrates were of the T-cell phenotype, CD3-positive and CD20-negative. CD4-positive cells predominantly among the T lymphocytes, although a few CD8-positive cells were also present.

Microscopically, no remnants of follicular B-cell lymphoma or any other malignancy were found.

The massive **myelo-radiculitis and vasculitis,** as often seen after these COVID-19 vaccinations, suggest a connection between the two corona COVID-19 vaccinations that took place and the death with a **probability bordering on certainty.**

2. Biopsies

43y / f / 1x Com
Skin-muscle biopsy from the lower extremity of a 43-year-old woman

C39B

Vaccination and disease history

The 43-year-old woman reports a COVID-19 infection in January 2021 and a COVID-19 vaccination with Comirnaty was received 6 months later.
1st vaccination on 8 July 2021 with Comirnaty FE7011, biopsy 254 days later
Subsequently, significant vaccination side effects of various kinds occurred, in particular circulatory disorders of the legs. Sonographically, a doubling of the vessel wall (wall thickening approx. 0.6 mm) was found in the dorsal popliteal artery.
In the distal anterior tibial artery and the posterior tibial artery, there was also an accentuation of the dorsal vessel walls with the described doubling of the vessel wall. A conspicuous feature was an intensified flow profile, which may indicate increased peripheral resistance in the wider capillary bed. A skin-subcutaneous muscle biopsy was taken from the lower leg for clarification. A primary examination of the biopsies was performed with the diagnosis: "Minimal superficial periadnexal dermatitis and minor superficial lymphocytic panniculitis. No evidence of malignancy".

Assessment of a skin-muscle biopsy

Macroscopic assessment: 7 x 5 mm measuring skin excisate with up to 10 mm wide adherent soft tissue.
Microscopic evaluation: 5 slides available, staining HE and Congo red. Immunohistology CD1a, SARS nucleocapsid, SARS spike protein. Regular, multilayered squamous epithelium with keratinisation on the surface. Pigmentation in the basal cell area. Increased dendritic, intraepithelial cells. Subepithelial smaller vessels with perivascular lymphocytic infiltrates. Slight thickening of the vessel wall and occasional hyalinisation. Occasionally also completely obliterated small arterioles. Tight fibrous tissue with inconspicuous skin appendages. In the subcutaneous fatty tissue, incision of a medium-sized artery with focal detachment of the endothelium and slight hyalinisation of the vessel wall. Furthermore, striated muscles of regular structure without inflammatory infiltrates.
In the Congo red staining, the slightly thickened vessel walls show a weak positive reaction for amyloid both subepidermally and more clearly in the fatty tissue.
Immunohistological imaging of the spike protein reveals positivity in the endothelia both in capillaries and in smaller arterioles. In addition, cytoplasmic expression in individual intraepithelial cells is conspicuously **(spike protein positive).**
In contrast, when the nucleocapsid was visualised, no such markings were found on any structure (nucleocapsid negative result).
With regard to the increased dendritic cells in the epithelium, which occasionally also express spike protein, an immunohistological examination for CD1a was also carried out. This reveals the so-called Langerhans cells, which perform an important immunological function in the epithelium. In fact, numerous Langerhans cells were

found to be positive, predominantly located suprabasally with some long dendritic projections extending below the stratum corneum layer. No positive reaction in the remaining tissue.

Diagnosis: Pronounced, partially obliterating inflammatory vasculopathy with amyloid deposits and positive expression of the spike protein.
Superficial periadnexal dermatitis with minor, predominantly lymphocytic panniculitis.
Proliferation of interepithelial Langerhans cells; foci with spike protein expression in the epidermis.

Epicrisis: The vascular changes are well compatible with the clinical findings of increased peripheral resistance in the capillary bed. The **amyloid deposits** in the vessel walls and the positive findings for the spike protein speak in favour of an association and probable causative role of the COVID-19-associated and vaccine-associated spike protein.
The perivascular, almost exclusively lymphocytic vasculitis and the significant proliferation of dendritic Langerhans cells in the epidermis suggest an ongoing immunological inflammatory process.
Myositis at the time of the biopsy could not be detected in the material taken from the surface. No evidence of malignancy.

Biopsy from the left calf (July 2023)
Question: Assessment of the elastic fibres
HE: Regularly stratified epidermis with slight orthokeratosis in the upper dermis. Capillaries with slight endothelial swelling and occasional pericapillary round cell infiltration.
Elastica: Significant **fragmentation** and clumping **of the elastic fibres.**
Berlin blue: Negative.
Spike: Spike protein positivity in the capillary endothelia and the surrounding fibrocytes.
Nucleocapsid: Negative.

Epicrisis: Obliterative microangiopathy with positivity of spike protein and spike-induced amyloid formation in the vessel walls. This means that there is a **high probability** of tissue damage induced by spike protein toxicity.

The patient also handed in a tube of her blood for examination at the institute in Reutlingen in October 2022. The section shows a fibrin thrombus without recognisable stratification. Such thrombi are often seen after COVID-19 vaccinations.

C113B

38y / m / 2x Com
Skin biopsy of a 38-year-old man

Vaccination and disease history

1st vaccination on 22 October 2021 with Comirnaty, batch number unknown
2nd vaccination on 10 March 2022 with Comirnaty, batch number unknown
Ten days after the 1st vaccination, cold symptoms, two days later PCR test positive. Bedridden for five days, fever up to 39.4 degrees Celsius with headache and sore throat, cough, lung pain, especially when coughing. Certificate of incapacity for work from the beginning of November. Lasting about 12 – 13 days.
Persistent complaints with diagnosis of "Long Covid": Stinging in the left chest, initially up to 12 times, now once a week regardless of movement or activity. Long-term headaches and lack of concentration.
After the 2nd vaccination on the following day, "sometimes extreme stinging" in the chest, emergency admission, but without pathological findings, was no longer taken seriously. Overall severe worsening of symptoms with increasing lack of concentration and headaches, feels foggy. Increasing forgetfulness. Stay in rehabilitation clinic from 14 March to 14 April 2022.

Consultant diagnosis

I: Epidermis preserved on the surface without basal cell damage and without inflammatory infiltrates. Immediately subepithelial vessels with marked endothelial swelling and focal perivascular inflammatory, predominantly lymphocytic infiltrates. Elastic destruction in deeper skin layers.
II: Subcutaneous fibrous tissue with elastic destruction.

Interpretation

Clear **vasculitis** immediately subepidermal with endothelial swelling and perivascular infiltrates predominantly by T lymphocytes, also mononuclear phagocytes. Clear **spike protein positivity** in the endothelia and inflammatory cells with negative nucleocapsid. No signs of spike protein in the epidermis and correspondingly normal epidermis corresponding to the absence of visible skin changes. **Destruction of elastic fibres** in the subepidermal connective tissue.
The overall histological findings are **almost certainly** indicative of COVID-19 vaccine-induced vasculitis. This is supported by the immunohistochemical spike protein detection with negative nucleocapsid.

C120B

63y / f / 1x Mod, 1x Com
Brain biopsy of a 63-year-old woman with right hemiparesis, gait ataxia, change in character

Vaccination and disease history

1st vaccination on 8 December 2021 with Moderna 3005690, biopsy 365 days later
2nd vaccination on 4 January 2022 with Comirnaty ACB4694, biopsy 338 days later

Previous history

Bipolar, affective disorder, diabetes mellitus, hypertension, malignant melanoma (first diagnosis 2010, localisation interclavicular, stage IA, pT1 Clark level III, 0.6 mm, resection)

Current medical history

June/July 2022: Hemiparesis on the right, gait ataxia, change in behaviour.
Admission to a regional psychiatric hospital.
Suspicion of cerebral metastases (left temporal, left basal ganglia area).
Transfer to an oncology department. No primary tumour found.
Initiation of radiotherapy. No biopsy due to the risky location.
November/December 2022: Acute deterioration with consciousness and motor disorders, psychosyndrome.
Admission to a regional psychiatric clinic.
cMRI shows massive increase in pathological brain findings.
7 December 2022: Stereotactic biopsy of the left thalamus.
Neuropathology: suspected vasculitis. Autoimmune diseases are not known in the woman.
Therapy with Cortisone and Cyclophosphamide leading to improvement.
End of December 2022: Suspicion of cerebral vasculitis.

Neuropathology

There are several lesions in the basal ganglia and in the thalamus on the left with rapid cognitive deterioration and clinical suspicion of a CNS lymphoma. There was also a history of radiotherapy.
Microscopically, we found no evidence of neoplasia and interpreted the tissue as **CNS** tissue with intramural inflammatory infiltrates, compatible **with vasculitis.** The reference centre also agreed with our interpretation and diagnosed a vascular inflammatory process, primarily vasculitis.

Consultation examination

A: In the overview, denser cell clusters around vessels. Overall, the cells in the brain substance also appear to be increased. Swollen vascular endothelia with dense inflammatory infiltrates.
B: Like A.
C: Like A; in addition a small focal necrosis in the brain substance.

Interpretation

In accordance with the findings of two different neuro-pathological clinics, we also see a profound and severe **vasculitis** with wall texture disorder, **amyloid-like deposits** in the vessel walls and residual vascular wall haemorrhages and perivascular haemorrhages. Impressive is the vascular and perivascular infiltration with dense aggregates of inflammatory cells, especially T lymphocytes (especially T8), fewer B lymphocytes, but abundant mononuclear phagocytes. Very few plasma

cells. These cells are also found scattered in the neighbouring brain tissue. Here very small necroses.
Immunohistological clear **positivity of the spike protein** in the area of the inflamed vessel walls and in inflammatory cells as well as in the adjacent brain tissue.
Such vasculitic/encephalitic changes are very frequently found in connection with COVID-19 vaccinations in varying degrees of severity, often minimal.
In view of the pronounced inflammatory changes and the clearly pronounced positivity of the spike protein in the lesions with a negative nucleocapsid, there is **almost certainly** a connection between the COVID-19 vaccinations that have taken place and the brain lesions.

70y / f / 2x Com **C140B**

Adrenal tumour biopsy of a 70-year-old woman

Vaccination and disease history

1st vaccination on 3 May 2021 with Comirnaty, biopsy 370 days later
2nd vaccination on 17 June 2021 with Comirnaty, biopsy 325 days later
High probability that a booster was also given once or twice.
Emergency admission in October 2021 after two falls at home, where she was found. In the past, frequent emergency admissions in an intoxicated state. Re-admission at the beginning of March 2022, this time with altered mental status and acutely ill appearance with fever, lactic acidosis and leucocytosis.
Sepsis with tissue infections on the right abdomen and bruises indicating past falls.
Admission due to sepsis, metabolic encephalopathy, dehydration and protein malnutrition.
April 2022 admission after collapse in septic state with altered mental status. Improvement after fluid and sepsis therapy.
After removal of the left kidney, initial post-operative recovery, followed by gradual deterioration and deep vein thrombosis.
Subsequently lethargic and somnolent with stable breathing. Severe protein malnutrition. Transfer to hospice service.
Final diagnosis at the end of April on transfer to hospice: Acute bacterial infection of the right flank (cellulitis) with metabolic acidosis, septic shock, encephalopathy and tumour in the left kidney. Pre-existing alcoholism. The patient died on 8 May 2022.

Consultant diagnosis

Anaplastic endocrine tumour.
Spike protein: Clear expression in the tumour cells, but tumour cells often give false positive signals in immunohistochemical examinations. Clear labelling of the vascular endothelia.
Nucleocapsid: No expression in the tumour cells. Vascular endothelia also negative.

Interpretation

In summary, the COVID-19 vaccination also led to spike expression in the tumour tissue and in the vessels of the tumour tissue. Whether or not COVID-19 vaccinations contribute causally to expression of tumour genesis and tumour progression cannot be assessed using pathohistological methods. In the future, epidemiological-statistical associations and possible molecular biological clues (e.g. spike protein effect on tumour genes and DNA repair mechanisms) must be sought.

3. Abortion

C157A

Abortion material embryo & placenta / 10th week of pregnancy 1x Astra, 2x Com in mother / 650 /616 /439

Immunisations of the parents

Mother

1st vaccination on 13 June 2021 with Astra, foetal death 650 days later
2nd vaccination on 17 July 2021 with Comirnaty, foetal death 616 days later
3rd vaccination on 10 January 2022 with Comirnaty, foetal death 439 days later

Father

1st vaccination on 13 June 2021 with Comirnaty EX3599
2nd vaccination on 22 July 2021 with Comirnaty FC3095
3rd vaccination on 15 January 2022 with Comirnaty ACB4447

After all three vaccination dates, a 'vaccine arm' appeared in the mother. The mother works on a COVID-19 ward.

The intrauterine foetal death occurred on 24 March 2023, the miscarriage about 3 weeks later.

Previous pregnancies

1. birth on 21 September 2018.
2. on 5 December 2021 miscarriage in the 6th week of pregnancy (between 2nd and 3rd COVID-19 vaccination).
3. on 20 February 2022 a pregnancy test was positive (after the 3rd vaccination), but the amniotic cavity was empty.
4. on 4 August 2022 miscarriage induction due to meningo-myelocele: On 29 May 2022 unremarkable prenatal test 11 + 1;

On 25 July 2022 2nd screening: lemon sign, banana sign, meningo-myelocele, Chiari II malformation (neural tube defect sign, spina bifida).

Course of pregnancy until intrauterine foetal death on 15 February 2023 (available material)

Gravida 5, Para 1, condition after 1x SPP (abortion), 3x miscarriage.
28 January 2023: Establishment of an intact intrauterine pregnancy (7 + 3).
24 March 2023: Diagnosis: Intrauterine foetal death.

13 April 2023: Fever, miscarriage (available examination material).
16 April 2023: Post curettage: (available examination material).

Consultation microscopic examination

I: Predominantly necrosis – possibly fetal tissue. In addition, endometrium with glands and cytogenic stroma.

II: Necroses and endometrium

Interpretation

Due to the **positive** detection of the **spike protein** with negative nucleocapsid in the endometrial tissue of the curettage, there is a **strong suspicion** that the abortion was caused by the COVID-19 vaccinations.

Summary of the findings

With regard to the groups described in the introduction (probability of a connection between death and COVID-19 vaccination), of the 89 autopsy cases

- 30 cases (34 % of the total number of deaths investigated) are assigned to group 1,
- 36 cases (40 % of the total number of deaths investigated) to group 2 and
- 23 cases (26 % of the total number of deaths investigated) to group 3.

This means that in almost three quarters of the autopsy cases analysed, the findings indicate that the death was almost certainly, very probably or probably related to the COVID-19 vaccination.

It was found that the *tissue damage was dependent on the number of COVID-19 vaccinations;* severe tissue damage was significantly more common in the deceased after multiple vaccinations than after a single vaccination.

It is important to point out that although the extent of damage in individual organs differed, the COVID-19 vaccination does not appear to lead to selective damage only in a few organs. Due to the mechanism of action of the mRNA, such damage was found in all organs examined. This lack of organ-specificity of the damage appears to be a characteristic of the mechanism of action of the immune response mediated by the mRNA or the autoimmune destruction of healthy endogenous cells triggered by it.

In 47 autopsy cases, i.e. in more than half of the cases, the cause of death was due to *myocarditis.* The deceased were aged between 16 and 94 years. The size of the myocarditis lesions varied. It was not uncommon for numerous incisions of the myocardium to be necessary to find the myocarditis foci.

Vasculitis was a very common finding. Mesaortitis with inflammation of the outer and middle wall layer of the aorta, which was rarely found in times before the COVID-19 vaccination, was found in 77 of 89 deaths. This inflammation was often concentrated around the vasa vasorum.

Another very striking finding was the fragmentation, clumping and *atrophy of the elastic fibres* both in the middle wall layer of the aorta and in other larger calibre vessels.

Other *vessel wall damage* such as media necrosis and oedematous swelling of the vessels in various organs could also be seen.

Immunohistochemical *detection of the spike protein* was frequently found in the blood and in the wall cells of blood vessels, especially capillaries. Here, destruction of the endothelia with exfoliation into the vessel lumen was frequently observed. It can be assumed that spike protein-containing blood plasma seeps through the resulting leaks into the neighbouring tissue, where it's toxicity attracts inflammatory cells and thus triggers severe inflammation. Spike protein was detectable in the endothelia of these supply vessels and in the surrounding macrophages. In the clearing of the affected blood vessels, thrombocytes partially agglutinated, leading to *thrombus formation.*

Another conspicuous finding in medium-sized and small blood vessels in various organs was irregular wall thickening. In most of these cases, a positive reaction could be detected with histochemical Congo red staining, proving *amyloidosis.* This pathological folding of large protein structures in the wall of these blood vessels, which cannot be broken down or absorbed by the body, leads to a permanent reduction in blood flow in the affected organ.

Due to the vessel wall damage, deposits and thrombus formation described above and *ischaemic phenomena* can often be seen in the organs.

In numerous cases, rod-shaped or needle-shaped crystalloide *deposits of uncertain origin* were found in the myocardium, pancreas, kidney, adrenal gland, lung, liver and/or skeletal muscle. The deposits were mostly concentrated in large quantities in tissue vacuoles, but spike protein was never detectable in them. They were analysed in several external institutes. Examination with the laser microscope showed an average length of 5 mm (variability from 1 to 8 mm) and an average width of 0.4 mm (variability from 0.2 to 0.6 mm). The ends were often corkscrew-shaped. The result of the energy dispersive X-ray spectroscopy more than strongly suggests organic material consisting of carbon and oxygen. There is no evidence of unorganic material. Using Raman spectrometry, the preliminary result was that it could be a crystal formation of cholesterol with bilirubin. Theoretically, it is therefore conceivable that the spike protein could destroy endothelia via atheroma beds of larger blood vessels, whereby the contents of the atheroma beds would enter the blood circulation and thus the organs.

The finding of *reduced spermatogenesis* in individual autopsy cases is also alarming, which is impressively demonstrated in the testicles of a 29-year-old in the findings section.

In the biopsies sent to the Institute by dermatologists or ENT specialists with various clinical diagnoses, lymphocytic vasculitis was found in the dermis and/or subcutis in almost all cases. The endothelia of the small blood vessels were exfoliated from the vessel wall and contained spike protein. The elastic fibres in the papillary zone appeared thinned or largely absent. This phenomenon could possibly explain the skin ageing frequently observed by clinicians in people vaccinated with COVID-19 agents.

Conclusion

An autopsy must be performed on every person who dies in connection with the COVID-19 vaccination.

Inquiring about the vaccination status, especially regarding mRNA vaccinations, should be part of every medical history. In addition to an external inspection of the deceased in order to detect and examine any vasculitic skin changes, the basic requirement for the post-mortem examiner is to open the three body cavities and carefully examine the findings. Histological examination of macroscopically clear findings such as aortic rupture, coronary thrombosis, myocardial infarction, cerebral haemorrhage and pulmonary embolism is also indicated in order to confirm or rule out a vasculitic component. Furthermore, numerous sections of the heart, preferably the entire heart, should be preserved in order to be able to reliably detect or rule out myocarditis. The sections should be analysed by experienced pathologists or forensic pathologists with experience in histology who are also familiar with the findings described in this atlas. Further special staining (e.g. Elastika-van-Gieson) and immunohistochemistry (e.g. spike protein and nucleocapsid) should be carried out. This is the only way to prove that it is a case of vaccine damage and not a so-called Long COVID case.

In any case, a summary should be made in which a statement is made on the probability of the connection between death and COVID-19 vaccination. The autopsy results must be published and made available to the relatives of the deceased.

All doctors must be made aware of the dangers of the new type of mRNA vaccination in order to stop further COVID-19 vaccinations of this kind and prevent so many people from suffering even more. There is a high risk that the damage described here could also be caused by other future mRNA-based vaccinations or other mRNA-based injections.

Some of the interpretations in this atlas are still preliminary; like any other new discovery, they should be discussed robustly and controversially. Silence, on the other hand, must come to an end!

Acknowledgements

We are extremely grateful to the lawyer Elmar Becker, to whom we owe the fact that the autopsy specimens and primary expertises of the deceased from the Institutes of Forensic Medicine or Clinical Pathology were made available for our consultative second opinions on behalf of the relatives of the vaccination victims.

Special thanks are due to the MWGFD, in particular Prof. Sucharit Bhakdi, for their great support, which was essential for the establishment and operation of the pathological institute in Reutlingen.

We would also like to thank Dr. Christian Fiala (Vienna, Austria) for his generous support. Without him, we would not have been able to continue our work in Reutlingen after the death of Prof. Burkhardt.

We are indebted to PD Dr. Norbert Schwarz for the registration and classification of the specimens submitted and the entire organisation of the laboratory work in Reutlingen. Without him, Prof. Burkhardt and Prof. Lang would not have been able to prepare their reports.

We would also like to thank the staff at the institute in Reutlingen, Oksana Faul, Ulrike Buschbacher and Enza Haider, whose hard work made it possible to further analyse the submitted material with special stains and immunohistochemical staining.

We would also like to thank the staff of the research institutes who examined the material, which had never been seen before, using methods that are not available in a pathological institute.

We are indebted to Prof. Dr. Ulrike Kämmerer (Würzburg, Germany) for the specificity study of the new antibodies on S1 protein and nucleocapsid using transfected cell cultures.

Of course, we would also like to thank our pathologist colleagues who were willing to be consulted; our special thanks go to Prof. Dr. Hubert Martin (Berlin, Germany) and Dr. Miklós Tarján (Falun, Sweden).

A very large, if not the largest, contribution to the completion of this atlas was made by all the generous donors who made it possible to sift through this extensive material again, digitise it and bring it into the form of this atlas: a very big thank you to Jan Veil and DDr. Christan Fiala.

Many thanks for the incredibly important help of our dear colleagues Dr. M.O. Gelin (Australia), Dr. Cordelia Kirchhoff-Stewens (Great Britain) and Dr. Paul Brandenburg (Germany) with the translation into English.

A very big thank you goes to Mrs Gabi Gerhardt (Germany), who did the typesetting of the book in English and to Gesa Schöning, who made it possible to publish this book in English in her publishing house.

Finally, our thanks go to all those who have encouraged us to compile this globally unique atlas.

About the authors

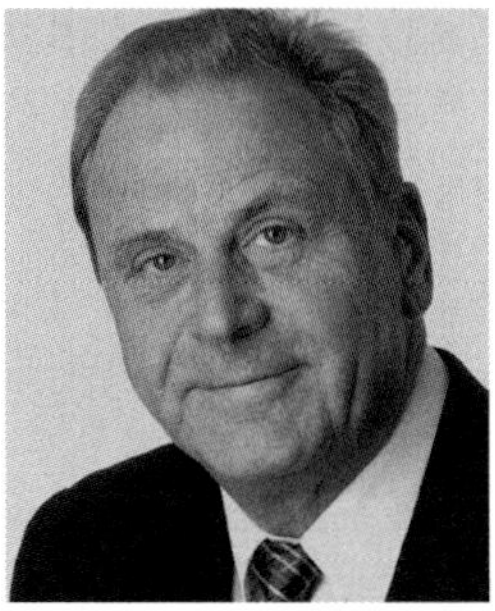

Prof. Dr. Arne Burkhardt was a German specialist in pathology and can look back on many years of teaching at the universities of Hamburg (Germany), Bern (Switzerland) and Tübingen (Germany) as well as visiting professorships/study visits in Japan (Nihon University), the USA (Brookhaven National Institute), Korea, Sweden, Malaysia and Turkey. He headed the Institute of Pathology in Reutlingen (Germany) for 18 years and subsequently worked as a pathologist in private practice. Prof. Burkhardt has published over 150 articles in specialist journals and as contributions to handbooks. He has also certified pathological institutes.

In recent years, he has primarily analysed tissue samples from deceased persons after COVID-19 vaccinations at his own institute in Reutlingen and prepared expert reports. These tissue samples were sent to him by forensic and pathological institutes from all over Europe. He showed an incredibly high level of commitment and published these findings in numerous international lectures.

Prof. Arne Burkhardt died suddenly in May 2023, and this book is dedicated to him.

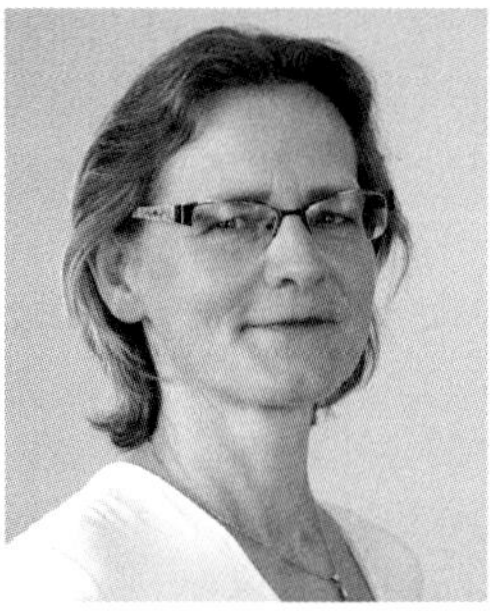

Dr. Ute Krüger is a German-trained, Swedish-based pathology specialist with 25 years of professional experience. She has worked as a consultant physician at the Swedish hospitals in Växjö and Kalmar for the past 18 years, primarily as a breast cancer specialist. For four years she also served as medical director of the pathology department in Växjö. During the last eight years of her career as a pathologist, she was involved in breast cancer research at the University of Lund alongside her clinical work at Kalmar Hospital. This resulted in several publications.

In the autumn of 2021, she noticed changes in the daily clinical examinations that seemed to be related to the COVID-19 vaccinations. She then coined the term 'turbo cancer'. In recent years, she has been in close contact and exchange with colleagues worldwide regarding changes after COVID-19 vaccination. She has helped to publish the novel findings after COVID-19 vaccinations made by Prof. Burkhardt and Prof. Lang in this book.

Due to the lack of response to her findings, she resigned from her position. She could not in an honest and sincere way continue to work as a pathologist in a system where the focus clearly is not on the health of patients. After several years of further training, she now works in her own holistic medical practice, specialising in disease prevention (www.active-health.se).

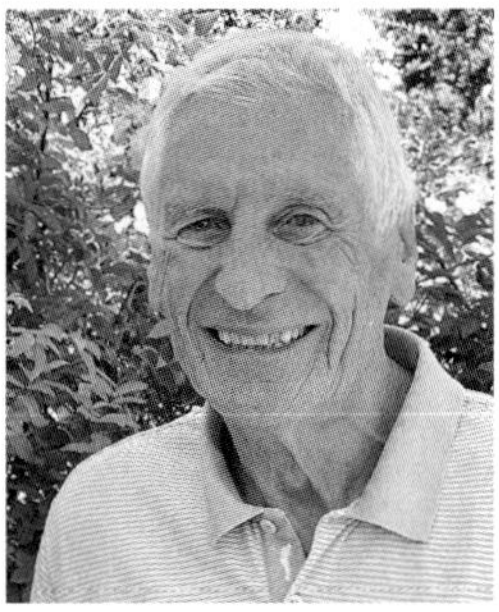

Prof. Dr. Walter Lang is a German specialist in pathology and worked at the Institute of Pathology at MHH Hannover Medical School (Germany) from 1968 to 1983, where he qualified as a professor and was awarded an adjunct professorship. His work and research focused on thyroid diseases (member of the EORCT and WHO – updated classification of thyroid tumours) and transplant pathology. In 1985, he founded a private institute for pathology in Hannover with consultative examinations for internal medicine clinics at universities, including the MHH and large clinics in northern Germany. from Saarland to Berlin in the fields of pneumology, liver diseases, bone marrow diseases and transplant pathology.

Since June 2021, he has worked with Prof. Burkhardt to provide expert opinions on damage caused by the COVID-19 vaccination.

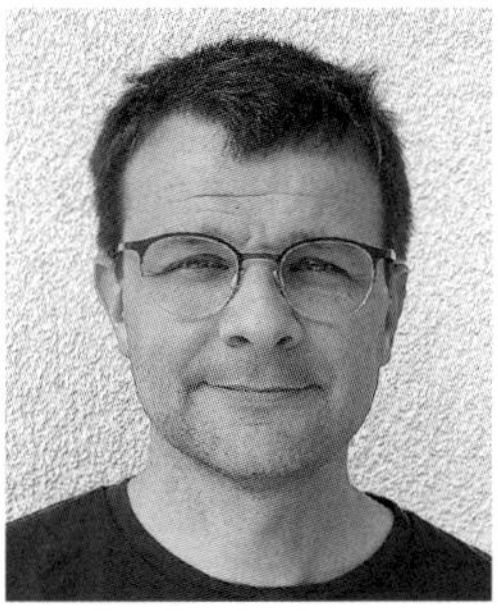

Dr. Michael Mörz is a German specialist in pathology. He completed his specialist training at the 'Georg Schmorl' Institute of Pathology at Dresden Municipal Hospital (Germany).

He joined the same centre as a senior physician in 2016. In recent years, he has worked intensively on the effects and side effects of SARS-CoV2 and gene-based vaccines. This has resulted in lectures and expert opinions as well as specialist articles in collaboration with other scientists.

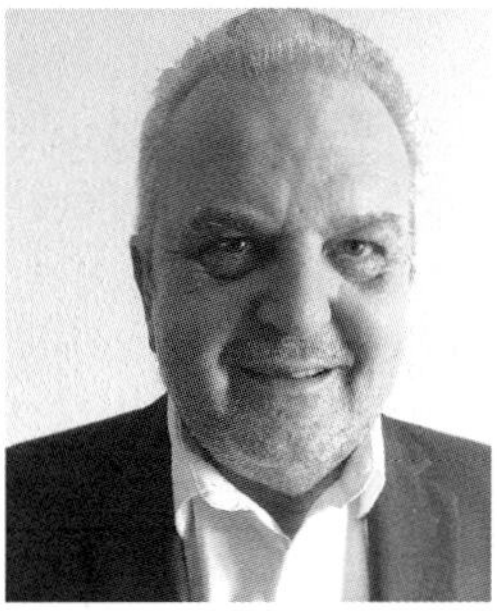

Prim. Dr. Helmut Luck is an Austrian specialist in pathology and microbiology. He began his professional career at the Kaiser Franz-Joseph Hospital in Vienna (Austria) and then went to the pathological institute of the Lillehammer Hospital in Norway for four years as a senior physician in 1999. He then worked for five years as a senior physician at the Institute of Pathology at Mistelbach Hospital in Austria. He then continued his career as an independent pathologist in private practice until 2013, when he took over as head of the pathological institute at Amstetten Regional Hospital in Austria.

In recent years, since the introduction of COVID-19 vaccinations, he has identified numerous changes in the examination material and has collaborated with many colleagues internationally.